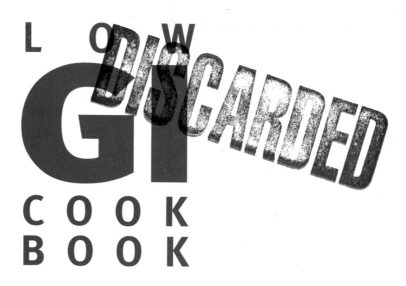

LOW GI COOKBOOK

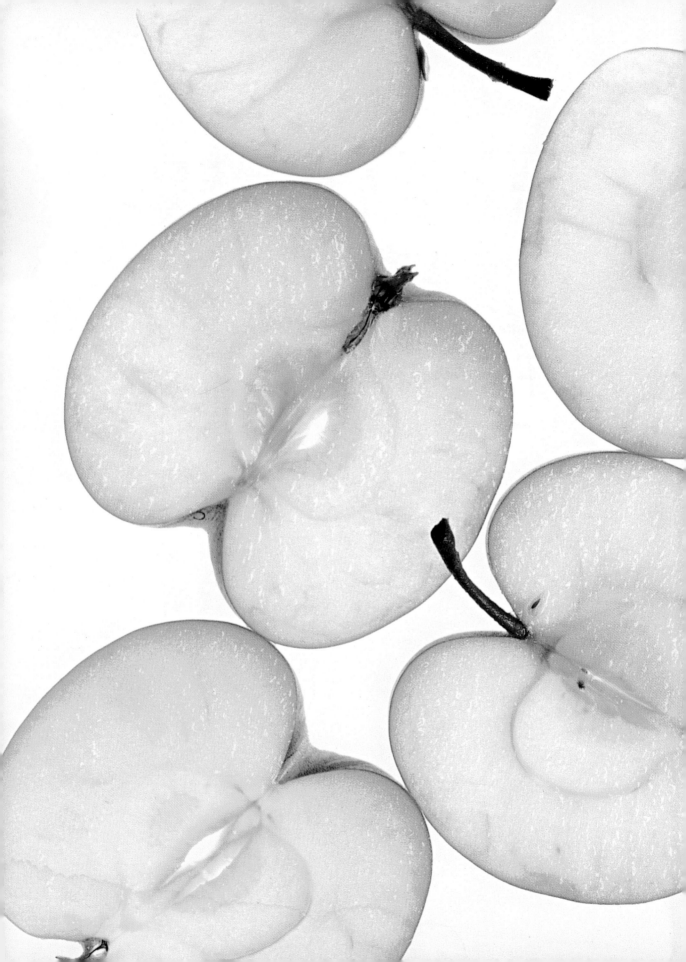

hamlyn

LOW GI COOKBOOK

**Over 80 delicious recipes to help
you lose weight and gain health**

Louise Blair

First published in Great Britain in 2005 by
Hamlyn, a division of Octopus Publishing Group Ltd
2–4 Heron Quays, London E14 4JP

Copyright © Octopus Publishing Group Ltd 2005

Distributed in the United States and Canada by
Sterling Publishing Co., Inc.
387 Park Avenue South, New York, NY 10016-8810

ISBN 0 600 61394 1
EAN 9780600613947

A CIP catalog record for this book is available from the British Library.

Printed and bound in China

10 9 8 7 6 5 4 3 2 1

NOTES

Standard level spoon measures are used in all recipes
1 tablespoon = one 15 ml spoon
1 teaspoon = one 5 ml spoon

Ovens should be preheated to the specified temperature. If using a fan-assisted oven, follow the manufacturer's instructions for adjusting the time and temperature. Broilers should also be preheated.

This book includes dishes made with nuts and nut derivatives. It is advisable for those with known allergic reactions to nuts and nut derivatives and those who may be potentially vulnerable to these allergies, such as pregnant and nursing mothers, invalids, the elderly, babies, and children, to avoid dishes made with nuts and nut oils. It is also prudent to check the labels of prepared ingredients for the possible inclusion of nut derivatives.

The FDA advises that eggs should not be consumed raw. This book contains some dishes made with raw or lightly cooked eggs. It is prudent for more vulnerable people such as pregnant and nursing mothers, invalids, the elderly, babies, and young children to avoid uncooked or lightly cooked dishes made with eggs.

Meat and poultry should be cooked thoroughly. To test if poultry is cooked, pierce the flesh through the thickest part with a skewer or fork — the juices should run clear, never pink or red.

All the recipes in this book have been analyzed by a professional nutritionist. The analysis refers to each serving.

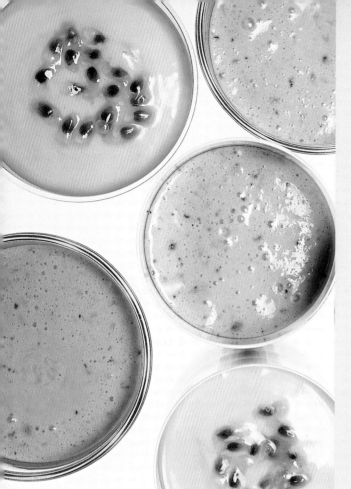

contents

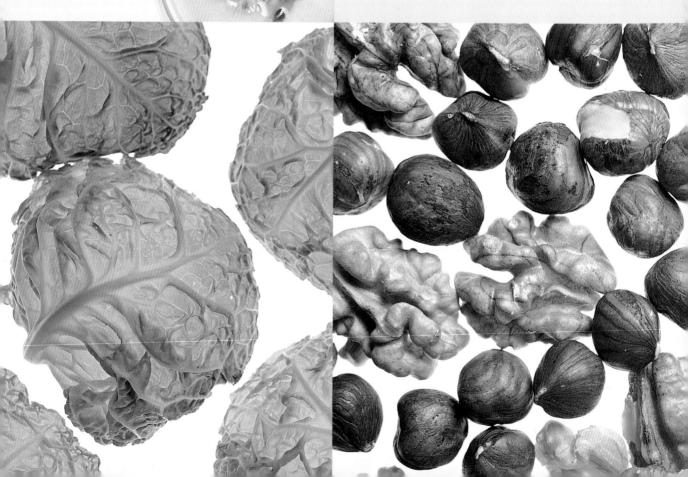

INTRODUCTION

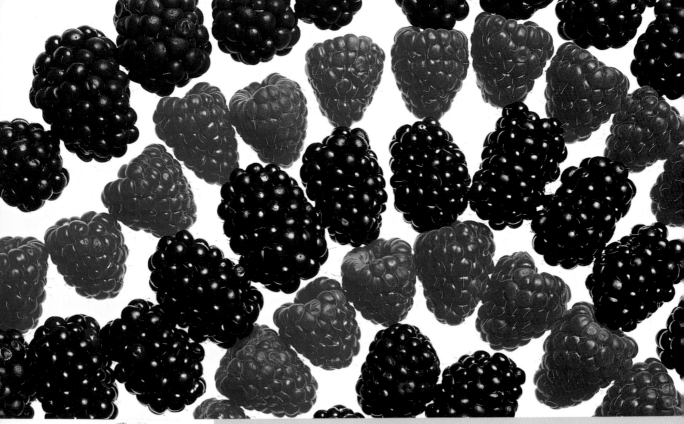

Over the following pages, you will learn about the benefits of switching to a low-GI diet. By sticking to a few simple rules, you can enjoy the many health rewards it can bring, without having to compromise on the taste or variety of your meals.

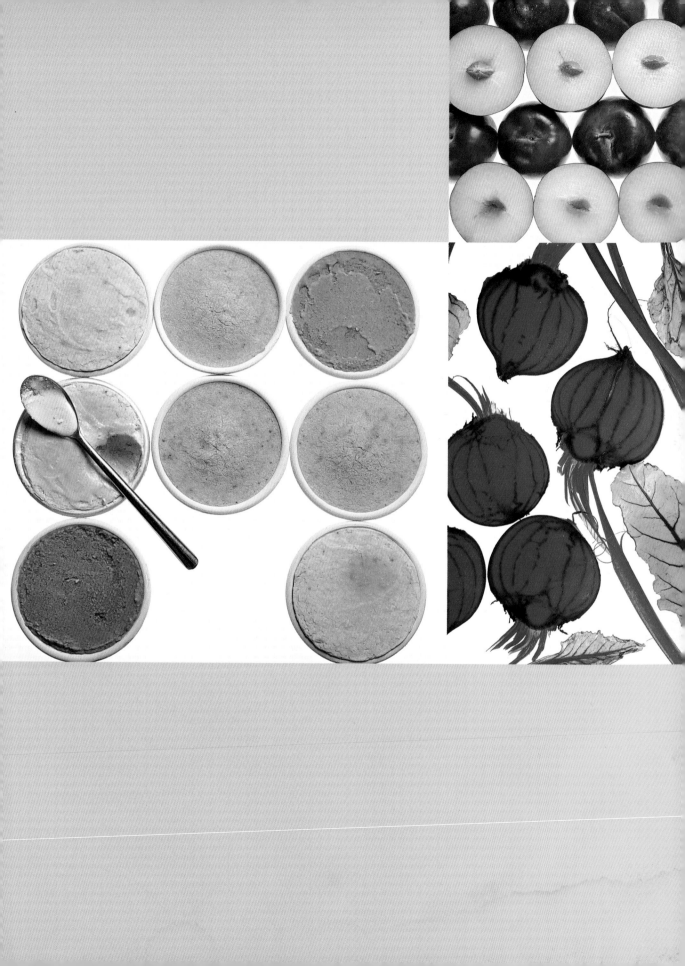

What is **GI**?

Put very simply, the glycemic index measures how the food you
eat reacts in your body. By following a low-GI diet, you choose
foods that create only a positive reaction.

The majority of the foods we eat come from one main food group—carbohydrates and, more specifically, white bread, potatoes, cakes, cookies, and sugary treats. While they taste good and are easy to eat, these foods create reactions in our bodies that put the entire system out of balance. The result of this imbalance is day-to-day problems such as fatigue, mood swings, and sugar cravings, plus an increased risk of a number of different health problems in the future. By basing your diet around the glycemic index of foods, you will stop all the confusion and allow your body to develop a sense of balance, without experiencing any harmful side effects.

Fueling your body

Your body requires a lot of energy to deal with all the stresses and strains of modern life and its preferred fuel is a sugar called glucose, which it makes from starches and sugars (carbohydrates) found in food. Glucose is made in the liver after the food has been digested in the stomach. The converted glucose is then sent to the body's cells where it is either burned immediately as we run, walk, or even think, or stored in the muscles and fat stores for later use. This happens with almost every food that contains carbohydrates, whether it is a plate of spinach or a plate of donuts. However, different foods affect the speed with which this reaction happens and, in very basic terms, the glycemic index is a measure of that speed. Foods with a high glycemic index (known as high-GI foods) are converted rapidly to glucose in the body, while foods with a low glycemic index (low-GI foods) are converted more slowly.

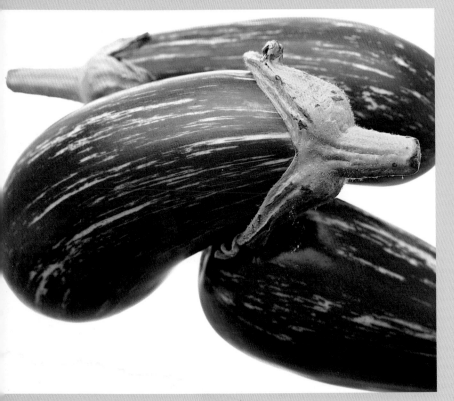

The missing **link**

A hormone called insulin provides the missing link in this process. When glucose is released into the bloodstream, insulin takes it to where it's needed. If the glucose is released slowly, moderate levels of insulin are released and have "time to think" about where that glucose is needed most and send it there. However, if high levels of glucose enter the bloodstream, the body panics—too much glucose can be harmful. To compensate, the body releases high levels of insulin, which quickly transfer the glucose to the fat stores where it can do no harm. If this happens too often, it can lead to weight gain as well as the cells that normally respond to glucose becoming resistant to its signals. This means that less glucose is taken to where it's needed, and it remains in the bloodstream, causing cell damage, which contributes to aging and clogging of the arteries.

About **turn**

By switching to a low-GI diet and ensuring you eat only foods that cause a gentle rise in glucose in your bloodstream, you can reverse this process and prevent a panic reaction in your system. The results can positively affect the condition and function of every part of your body, from your heart to your skin, and will boost weight loss.

All foods are **not equal**

When choosing a GI eating plan, it is important that you know which foods are best to choose. There are six main elements that determine the GI of a food:

❶ Does it contain carbohydrate?
Pure protein foods such as meat, fish, poultry, and eggs, and pure fats such as oils, butter, and margarine, contain no carbohydrate, so the effect they have on glucose production is negligible. These foods are therefore low GI.

❷ How much starch does it contain, and in what form?
Starch is the easiest ingredient for our body to turn into glucose. In raw foods, where this starch is generally in compact particles, the body finds it difficult to break down. However, if these particles are disturbed (for example, milling into flour), the body finds it easier to digest them and therefore turns them into glucose faster.

❸ How much fiber does it contain?
Fiber makes the body break food down more slowly, which is one of the reasons why beans and lentils (which are wrapped in a fibrous shell) have such a low GI.

❹ What kind of sugar does it contain?
There are four main types of sugar. Foods high in glucose (such as sports drinks) need no

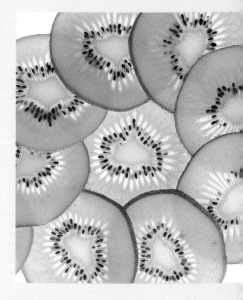

conversion, so they raise blood sugar rapidly, while fructose (the sugar in fruit) and lactose (the main sugar in dairy products) convert slowly. This gives the majority of foods containing fructose or lactose a low GI. The fourth sugar, sucrose, has a medium GI.

❺ Does it contain fat?
Fat has no effect on glucose itself, but it does slow the speed of food from the stomach to the liver, in turn slowing glucose production.

❻ How acidic is it?
Citrus fruits are an example of foods that contain acid ingredients, in this case citric acid. Other acidic ingredients include lactic acid in milk products. Acidity slows a food's progress through the system, and therefore the rate at which it converts into glucose.

GI facts about **carbohydrates**

If you follow a GI diet, the biggest changes you will probably make to your regular diet are to the following six foods: bread, breakfast cereal, grains, pasta, potatoes, and rice. It is often these foods that make up the majority of our diet and they are also the easiest to convert into glucose. Don't panic though; the low-GI diet doesn't ban starchy carbohydrates. The idea is to switch your choices to those with the lowest impact on your blood sugar levels.

Bread

Many of us tend to eat a lot of bread. This is fine as long you opt for low-GI breads that are high in fiber—whole wheat or whole grain are best, as the hard husk around the grains slows glucose conversion. Breads made from an ingredient with a lower GI than wheat are also a good choice. These include soy bread and rye bread.

Breakfast cereals

It's important to eat breakfast as it prevents you getting hunger pangs that lead you to eating less-nutritious snacks mid-morning. However, a high-GI breakfast cereal is just as likely to leave you hungry as having no breakfast at all. You should avoid cereals that have been processed or have high levels of added sugar or honey, and instead go for high-fiber cereals such as bran, or opt for traditional oatmeal.

Grains

Grains are subject to minimal processing, so most have a low GI. They are also generally high in essential B vitamins and vital minerals such as magnesium or phosphorus. Barley, buckwheat, bulgur wheat, millet, and quinoa (which is actually a fruit) are all low GI, while couscous is medium GI. They can all be used instead of potatoes or rice as a side dish and are also very easy and quick to prepare.

Pasta

Surprisingly, almost all pastas are low-GI foods. This is because the flour used to make them (durum wheat) contains protein, which slows its digestion. The starch particles in pasta are left fairly intact, which also slows things down. The problem with pasta is that we generally eat much larger portions than recommended, thereby increasing the amount of glucose produced. It's best to eat pasta "al dente"—the softer the pasta, the higher its GI rating. The exception is gluten-free pasta. This is made with wheat-free flour, so doesn't have the protein protection provided by durum wheat.

Noodles

Some noodles are made from a more glutinous form of wheat flour, so are best avoided. However, glass (bean thread) noodles, cellophane noodles, and harusame noodles are made of beans and have a very low GI rating.

Potatoes

Potatoes may be a great source of vitamin C, potassium, and the anti-aging nutrient glutathione, but they score badly on the GI plan. This is believed to be due to their high starch content, which increases if new potatoes are left on the plant to grow. In fact, new potatoes are the only potatoes to have a low GI, so choose these wherever possible, or swap potatoes for another, low-GI, carbohydrate. The other option is to use sweet potatoes, which have a medium GI and can be prepared in much the same way as regular potatoes.

Rice

The GI content of rice is dependent upon which type of starch it contains—amylose, which is tightly bonded together, or amylopectin, which is more branched out. Rices high in amylose have a lower GI.

Carbohydrate snacks

Most snacks have a high GI and even savory snacks can raise glucose levels too quickly. However, snacking is actually encouraged on a low-GI diet, as eating a small meal or snack every two hours keeps blood sugar levels even more stable than eating three large meals a day. Try nuts, seeds, fruit, yogurt—or a little chocolate. Yes, you may be surprised to learn that chocolate has a low GI, due to a high concentration of dairy products, a high fat content, and also its sucrose content, which converts into glucose at a slow rate.

GI facts about **fruit** and **vegetables**

Fruit

As a general rule, fruit is a low-GI food. The main sugar in many fruits is fructose, which has to be converted into glucose before it can be used by the body, thus preventing the sudden peak in blood sugar that can cause rapid insulin release.

What affects the GI of a fruit?

Acidity Generally, the more acidic a particular fruit is, the lower its glycemic index.

Fiber content Fruits with the highest soluble fiber content (such as apples and pears) are those with the lowest GI.

Fructose content Most fruit contains a mixture of three sugars: fructose, sucrose, and glucose. The more fructose (and less glucose) a fruit contains, the lower its GI.

Processing Canning softens the fibrous strands in fruit, making it easier to break down and slightly increasing the rate at which glucose is created. Fruit is also often canned in syrup, which can contain fast-release sugars, and raises GI from low to medium. Fruit juice also has a higher GI, as the fiber has been removed.

Vegetables

Like fruit, the majority of vegetables are low-GI foods. Despite the fact that many are classed as carbohydrate foods, the actual amount of carbohydrates they contain is very small. As well as this, most vegetables are very high in fiber, which is a GI inhibitor. There are some exceptions to this, such as starchy root vegetables (beets, parsnips, and rutabaga), or sweet vegetables (pumpkin), which are medium- or high-GI foods. This doesn't mean you should never eat these—as long as you keep portions moderate and don't eat them at every meal, there's no reason to entirely ban high-GI vegetables from your diet.

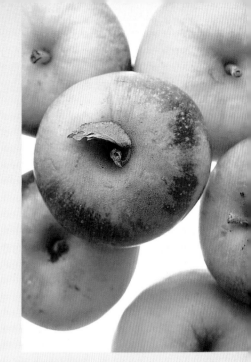

GI facts about **protein** foods

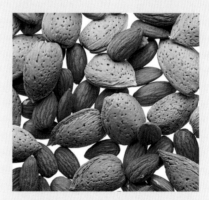

Pure protein foods contain no carbohydrate and so have a low GI. However, foods that contain high levels of protein, but also some level of carbohydrate, have a higher GI rating.

Legumes A diet containing regular servings of legumes such as beans and lentils has been shown to lead to lower cholesterol levels, and to help balance hormones in women, possibly reducing the risk of breast cancer—so we should all be eating more of them. Most legumes have a low GI due to the fibrous coating around them, which slows conversion.

Dairy products Many dairy products contain the sugar lactose, which is converted into glucose in the body. However, these sugars are converted slowly, meaning that dairy products such as milk, cheese, and yogurt are low-GI foods.

Nuts and seeds The combination of protein and fats gives nuts and seeds their low GI. Some nutritionists describe seeds as a superfood and they can easily be eaten by the handful as a snack or sprinkled over salads. Remember too that spreads and dips made from nuts and seeds, such as peanut butter and tahini, will also have a low GI.

When **low**-GI meets **high**

No one wants to eat the same foods every day and the great thing about the GI eating plan is that no food is completely banned. There are, however, a few simple rules to follow when you eat a high-GI food.

The **rules**

❶ When you eat a high-GI food, watch your portion size. The more you eat of a food, the greater amounts of glucose will be produced, so if you eat less, you create less.

❷ Every time you eat a high-GI food, you should accompany it with at least two low-GI foods of the same or a larger quantity to lower the average GI of the meal. Ideally, one of the accompanying foods should be a protein food and the other should be fruit or vegetables. So, for example, if you have 1 oz or 1 cup of high-GI cornflakes for breakfast, accompany this with ⅓ cup of skim milk and a sliced fresh peach.

❸ Avoid eating more than one high-GI food or two medium-GI foods in any one day—and, if at all possible, eat fewer than this. By sticking to this simple approach, you will be giving your body the chance to really get back into balance.

❹ Try to add something acidic to your meal wherever possible. In the same way that acid integrated into a food slows its conversion to glucose, so does acid added to a high-GI food. So, for example, you could eat half a grapefruit with a high-GI breakfast or accompany a main meal containing rice with a fresh side salad, topped with a vinaigrette dressing.

Low-GI portions for high-GI foods

Potatoes 3½ oz
Rice 3 oz or ½ cup cooked weight, roughly 1 tablespoon or 1 oz dried
Bread 1–2 slices
Breakfast cereals 1 oz or 1 cup
Root vegetables 3½ oz
Popcorn and pretzels 1 oz

10 **reasons** to eat low-GI foods

❶ Your heart will thank you. According to research conducted at Harvard University, women with a high intake of refined carbohydrates have 10 percent less good cholesterol in their bloodstream. Good cholesterol keeps the heart healthy.

❷ High levels of homocysteine are linked to heart problems and the development of Alzheimer's disease in later life. By taking simple measures, such as swapping rice for whole grains, your levels of homocysteine can fall dramatically.

❸ A diet rich in high-GI foods may increase the risk of breast cancer. The reason is that high insulin levels trigger an increase in insulin-like growth hormones, which can encourage breast cancer cells to grow.

❹ Health experts recommend eating about 1 oz of fiber a day. A high-fiber content is a contributing factor in making a food low GI, so by increasing your intake of low-GI foods, you are more likely to achieve this. Increased fiber consumption will boost weight loss, because fiber helps sweep fat calories out of the system.

❺ Many dermatologists believe that refined carbohydrates trigger inflammation of the skin, which can affect the collagen and elastin fibers that keep skin firm. So, by cutting sugary foods out of your diet, you will help yourself to look younger.

❻ Reducing insulin levels can help acne and oily skin. High insulin levels lead to the release of higher levels of androgens in the system, which trigger excess sebum production.

❼ According to the World Health Organization, the number of people suffering from diabetes will double by the year 2030. Switching to low-GI diets could cut the number of potential sufferers dramatically. A low-GI diet can also help existing diabetes sufferers to control their condition more effectively, as it can help keep blood glucose levels more stable.

❽ A low-GI diet can reduce the risk of stroke. Women who switched just one serving of refined carbohydrates to whole grains each day cut their risk of stroke by 40 percent, say researchers at Harvard University.

❾ Sugary foods attack your immune system. When fighting illness, the average white blood cell can destroy about 14 germs in an hour. However, when exposed to 3½ oz of sugar, that number falls to 1.4 germs per hour, and stays that way for two hours. Low-GI eating will potentially cut the risks of ailments such as colds and flu.

❿ Many exercisers think they need high-sugar bursts to fuel their bodies, but in fact sticking to a low-GI diet throughout the majority of training actually increases endurance.

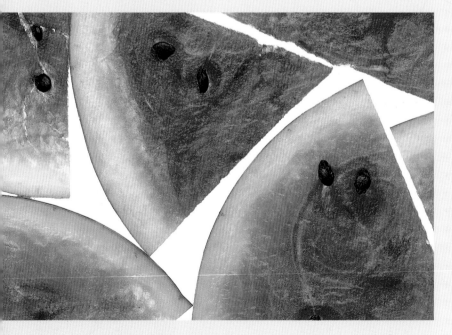

START THE DAY

From a quick bite to a hearty meal, a good breakfast really does set you up for the day ahead. There's plenty here to suit every appetite and time constraint.

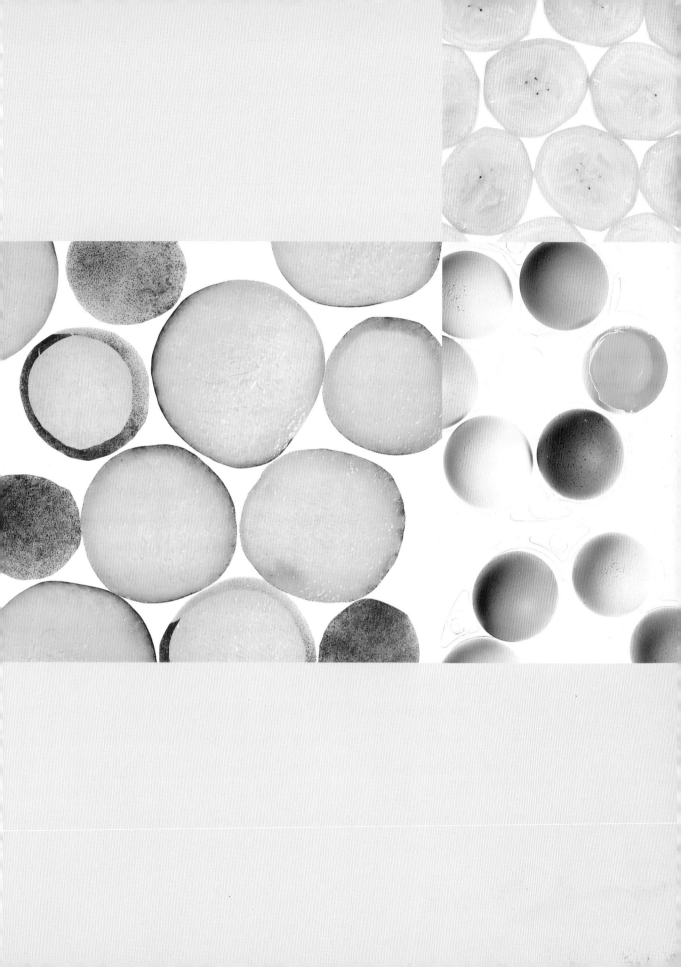

wild mushroom omelet

preparation: 10 minutes | **cooking:** 20 minutes | **serves:** 4

2 tablespoons butter

7 oz wild mushrooms, trimmed and sliced

8 large eggs, beaten

2 tablespoons chopped parsley

2 oz Gruyère cheese, grated

pepper

whole wheat or whole grain toast, to serve

1 Melt a little of the butter in an omelet pan, add the mushrooms, and sauté for 5–6 minutes until cooked and any moisture has evaporated. Remove the mushrooms from the pan and set aside.

2 Melt a little more butter in the same pan and add one-quarter of the beaten egg. Season well with pepper and stir with a wooden spoon, bringing the cooked egg to the center of the pan and allowing the runny egg to flow to the edge and cook.

3 When there is only a little liquid egg left, sprinkle over a few mushrooms and some of the parsley and Gruyère, fold the omelet over, and tip on to a warm serving plate. Repeat with the remaining ingredients. Serve with whole wheat or whole grain toast.

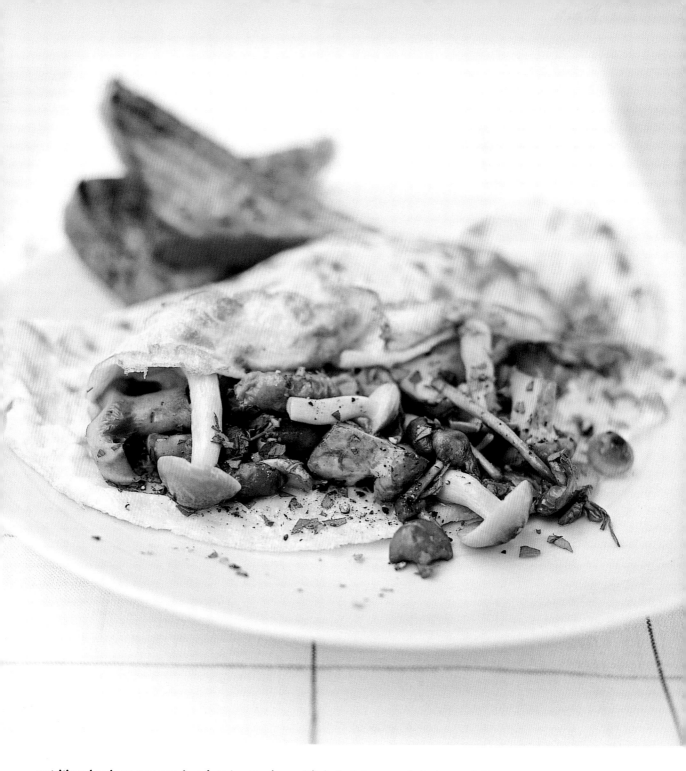

nutritional values per serving | Cals **282 (1172 kj)** | Protein **19 g** | Carb **0 g** | Fat **23 g**

easy corned beef hash

preparation: 10 minutes | **cooking:** 10 minutes | **serves:** 4

1 teaspoon olive oil

1 onion, chopped

11½ oz cooked new potatoes, coarsely chopped

11½ oz corned beef, coarsely chopped

1 tablespoon chopped parsley

Worcestershire sauce, to taste

pepper

thick whole wheat or whole grain toast, to serve

1 Heat the oil in a large, nonstick skillet. Add the onion and fry for 2–3 minutes until softened.

2 Add the potatoes and corned beef and continue to fry for 6–7 minutes, turning the mixture occasionally so that parts of it become crisp.

3 Stir through the parsley, then season to taste with Worcestershire sauce and pepper. Serve with thick whole wheat or whole grain toast. For a change, you could also serve the hash topped with a poached egg.

nutritional values per serving | Cals **277** (1162 kJ) | Protein **25 g** | Carb **19 g** | Fat **12 g**

creamy herby scrambled eggs on rye

preparation: 5 minutes | **cooking:** 5 minutes | **serves:** 4

8 large eggs

4 tablespoons milk

1 tablespoon polyunsaturated margarine

2 tablespoons light cream cheese

2 tablespoons chopped mixed tender herbs (such as parsley, oregano, and chives)

salt, if liked, and pepper

4 thick slices of rye bread, to serve

1 In a bowl, beat the eggs and milk together and season with salt, if liked, and pepper. Heat the margarine in a nonstick skillet, add the egg mixture, and stir constantly with a wooden spoon for a few minutes until the eggs are softly set.

2 Remove the pan from the heat and stir in the cream cheese and herbs, then serve on thick slices of rye bread.

nutritional values per serving | Cals **300 (1252 kJ)** | Protein **19 g** | Carb **15 g** | Fat **19 g**

pear pancakes

preparation: 10 minutes | **cooking:** 20 minutes | **serves:** 4 (makes 12 small pancakes)

¼ cup polyunsaturated margarine, melted

⅓ cup self-rising flour

⅓ cup whole wheat self-rising flour

3 tablespoons oatmeal

1 tablespoon caster sugar

2 eggs, lightly beaten

generous 1 cup buttermilk

milk, for thinning (optional)

oil, for brushing

6 pears, peeled, cored, and chopped

pinch of ground cinnamon

1 tablespoon water

1 In a bowl, beat the margarine, flours, oatmeal, sugar, eggs, and buttermilk together until smooth, adding a little milk if the mixture looks very thick.

2 Brush a nonstick skillet with a little oil and heat. Add a ladleful of batter to the pan and cook for 2 minutes on each side until golden. Remove the pancake from the pan and keep warm. Repeat with the remaining batter mixture.

3 Meanwhile, place the pears and cinnamon in a small pan with the water. Cover and cook gently for 2–3 minutes until just tender. Serve the pancakes with the cooked pears.

tip

If you can't find buttermilk, mix equal quantities of plain yogurt and skim milk together.

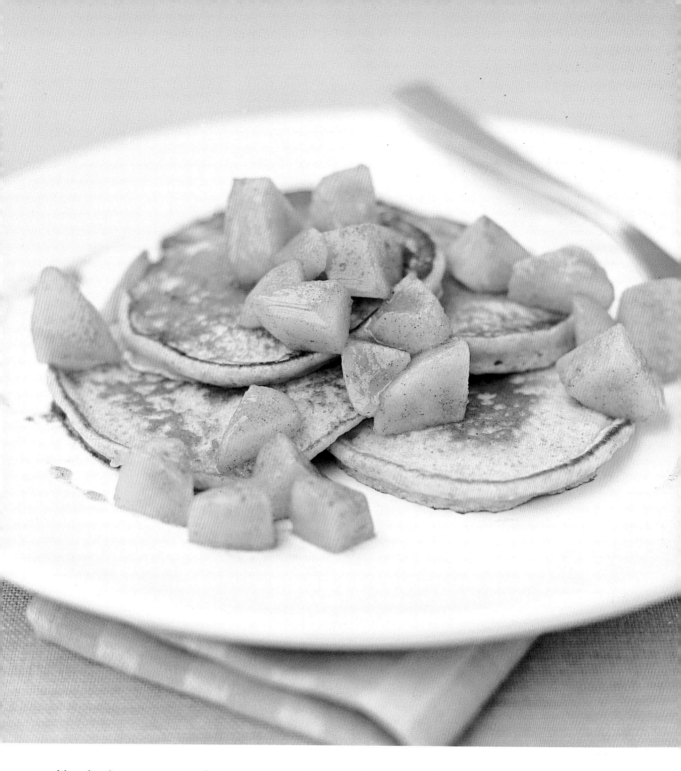

nutritional values per serving | Cals **378 (1585 kj)** | Protein **10 g** | Carb **52 g** | Fat **16 g**

buckwheat pancakes with banana and cream cheese

preparation: 10 minutes | **cooking:** 10 minutes | **serves:** 4 (makes 4 large or 8 small pancakes)

⅓ cup all-purpose flour

⅓ cup buckwheat flour

1¼ cups skim milk

1 egg, beaten

oil, for brushing

generous ⅓ cup light cream cheese

4 small bananas, sliced

1 Sift the flours together into a bowl, tipping any bran in the strainer back into the bowl. Whisk the milk and egg together and gradually add to the flour, beating to form a smooth batter.

2 Brush a nonstick skillet with a little oil and heat. Add a ladleful of batter to the pan and cook for 1–2 minutes on each side until golden. Remove the pancake from the pan and keep warm. Repeat with the remaining batter mixture.

3 Smooth a little cream cheese over each pancake and top with some sliced banana. Fold in half and serve.

nutritional values per serving | Cals **276 (1160 kj)** | Protein **10 g** | Carb **43 g** | Fat **8 g**

porridge with apricot purée

2⅓ cups rolled oats

3 cups skim milk or water

2 teaspoons brown sugar

generous 1 cup no-soak dried apricots

1¼ cups orange juice

1 Place the oats, milk or water, and sugar in a pan and bring to a boil. Reduce the heat and simmer for about 10 minutes until the oats are softened and the required consistency is reached.

2 Meanwhile, place the apricots and orange juice in a separate pan and bring to a boil. Reduce the heat and simmer for 10 minutes. Transfer to a food processor or blender and process until smooth. Serve the purée over the porridge.

tip

As an alternative you could serve the porridge with poached fruit of your choice, such as cherries or plums.

nutritional values per serving | Cals **344 (1460 kj)** | Protein **14 g** | Carb **66 g** | Fat **5 g**

blueberry, peach, and citrus salad with whole grain yogurt

preparation: 10 minutes | **serves:** 4

1⅓ cups blueberries

2 oranges, segmented

2 grapefruits, segmented

2 peaches, halved, pitted, and sliced

¼ cup toasted whole grains

scant 1¼ cups plain yogurt

2 teaspoons maple syrup

1 Divide the prepared fruit between 4 bowls. Mix the remaining ingredients together and spoon over the fruit. Serve.

tip

If you can't find whole grains in your local health-food store or supermarket, you can replace them with toasted mixed nuts.

Oranges are a good source of **folates**. These are essential to a baby's development in the womb and for the formation of red blood cells in adults. All citrus fruits are **high in vitamin C** as well, which **helps fight infection**.

nutritional values per serving | Cals **183 (775 kj)** | Protein **7 g** | Carb **38 g** | Fat **1 g**

toasted fruity granola

preparation: 10 minutes I **serves:** 4

1¼ cups jumbo oats, toasted

3 tablespoons wheatgerm

1 oz toasted mixed seeds (such
as pumpkin, sunflower, and
sesame)

1 tablespoon hazelnuts, toasted
and coarsely chopped

generous ¼ cup no-soak dried
apricots

⅓ cup dried cranberries

3 dried figs, chopped

lowfat milk, to serve

1 Simply combine all the
ingredients in a large mixing
bowl and serve in bowls with
lowfat milk.

tip

This granola is also
delicious served with
plain yogurt and
chopped fresh fruit, such
as pears and apples, or
summer berries.

nutritional values per serving I Cals **293 (1237 kj)** I Protein **9 g** I Carb **48 g** I Fat **9 g**

dried fruit compote

preparation: 5 minutes, plus standing | **cooking:** 10 minutes | **serves:** 4

3 cups mixed no-soak dried fruit of your choice (such as apricots, figs, prunes, and cranberries)

1 cinnamon stick

1 star anise

2 cardamom pods

generous ¾ cup water

generous ⅓ cup apple juice

plain yogurt, to serve

1 Place all the ingredients in a pan and bring to a boil. Reduce the heat, cover, and simmer for 10 minutes. Remove from the heat and set aside for at least 30 minutes. Serve with plain yogurt.

nutritional values per serving | Cals **218 (930 kJ)** | Protein **4 g** | Carb **51 g** | Fat **1 g**

super smoothies

basic smoothie mixture

preparation: 5 minutes | **serves:** 1

1 small banana

⅔ cup lowfat plain yogurt

¾ cup skim milk

few drops of vanilla extract

nutritional values per serving
I Cals **226 (956 kj)** | Protein **15 g** | Carb **40 g** | Fat **2 g**

1 Whiz all the ingredients together in a food processor or blender until smooth. Serve in a tall glass.

tropical fruit smoothie

1 Add the flesh of ½ ripe mango to the Basic Smoothie Mixture ingredients. Whiz all the ingredients together in a food processor or blender until smooth, then stir through the flesh of 1 passion fruit. Serve in a tall glass.

nutritional values per serving
I Cals **276 (1160 kj)** | Protein **16 g** | Carb **51 g** | Fat **2 g**

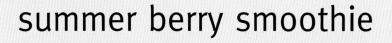

summer berry smoothie

1 Add ½ cup mixed summer berries (thawed if frozen) to the Basic Smoothie Mixture ingredients. Whiz all the ingredients together in a food processor or blender until smooth. Serve in a tall glass.

nutritional values per serving
| Cals **247 (1036 kj)** | Protein **16 g** | Carb **43 g** | Fat **2 g**

apple and oat smoothie

1 Add 1 peeled, cored, and chopped apple, 2 teaspoons clear honey, and 2 tablespoons granola to the Basic Smoothie Mixture ingredients. Whiz all the ingredients together in a food processor or blender until smooth. Serve in a tall glass.

nutritional values per serving
| Cals **415 (1750 kj)** | Protein **19 g** | Carb **80 g** | Fat **4 g**

QUICK-FIX LUNCHES

Lunch on the go doesn't have to mean a sandwich. These recipes are all quick to prepare, or they can be cooked while you're doing other things. Being busy is all the more reason to have a lunch that you can look forward to.

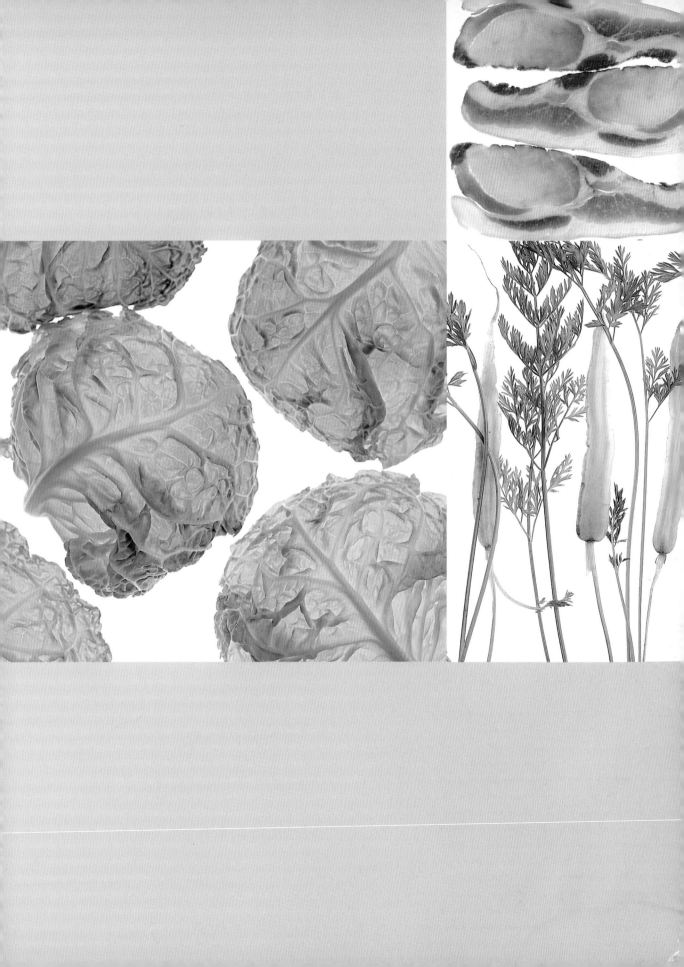

summer vegetable soup

preparation: 10 minutes | **cooking:** 15 minutes | **serves:** 4

1 teaspoon olive oil

1 leek, finely sliced

1 large potato, chopped

14½ oz mixed summer vegetables (such as peas, asparagus, fava beans, and zucchini)

2 tablespoons chopped mint

3½ cups Vegetable Stock (see below)

2 tablespoons lowfat sour cream

salt, if liked, and pepper

1 Heat the oil in a medium pan, add the leek, and fry for 3–4 minutes until softened.

2 Add the vegetables to the pan with the mint and the stock and bring to a boil. Reduce the heat and simmer for 10 minutes.

3 Transfer the soup to a food processor or blender and process until smooth. Tip back into the pan with the sour cream and season with salt, if liked, and pepper. Heat through and serve.

vegetable stock

preparation: 10 minutes | **cooking:** 1½ hours | **makes:** about 1 quart

1 tablespoon olive oil

1 onion, chopped

1 carrot, chopped

4 celery stalks, chopped

any vegetable trimmings (such as celery tops, onion skins and tomato skins)

1 bouquet garni

7 cups water

salt and pepper

1 Heat the oil in a large pan, add the vegetables and trimmings, and fry for 2–3 minutes. Add the bouquet garni and season well with salt and pepper. Add the water and bring to a boil. Reduce the heat and simmer gently for 1½ hours. Strain.

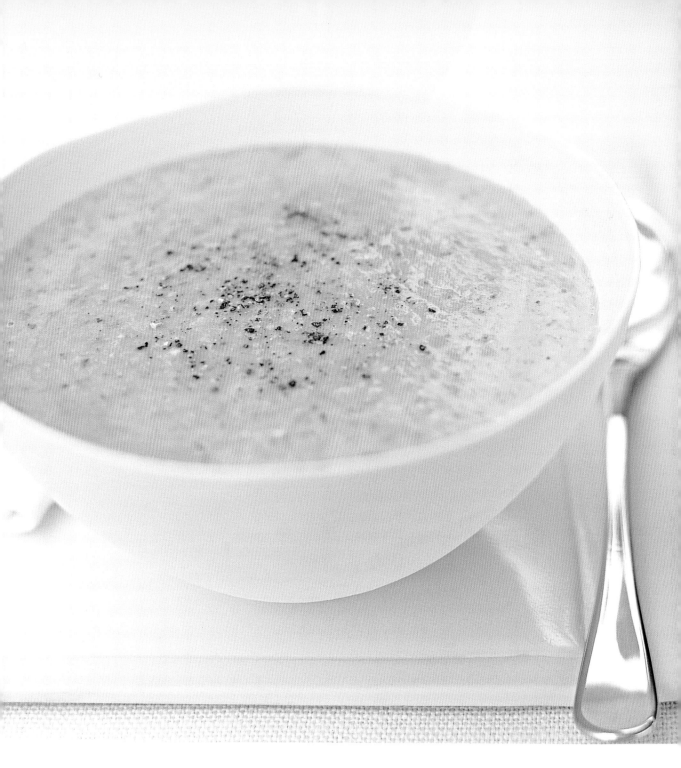

nutritional values per serving | Cals **136 (566 kj)** | Protein **6 g** | Carb **17 g** | Fat **5 g**

corn chowder

preparation: 15 minutes | **cooking:** 25 minutes | **serves:** 4

1 teaspoon olive oil

1 onion, chopped

14½ oz potatoes, chopped

2½ cups Vegetable Stock (see page 32)

1¼ cups milk

1 bay leaf

11 oz can corn kernels, drained

2 large tomatoes, chopped

2 tablespoons chopped parsley

salt, if liked, and pepper

1 Heat the oil in a medium pan, add the onion, and fry for 2–3 minutes until beginning to soften. Add the potatoes and continue to fry for 2 minutes, then add the stock, milk, and bay leaf. Bring to a boil, then reduce the heat and simmer gently for 15 minutes.

2 Add the corn and tomatoes and continue to simmer for 5 minutes, then remove the bay leaf. Transfer the soup to a food processor or blender and process until smooth. Return to the pan with the parsley and season with salt, if liked, and pepper. Heat through and serve.

nutritional values per serving | Cals **265 (1123 kj)** | Protein **8 g** | Carb **50 g** | Fat **5 g**

chicken and pearl barley broth

preparation: 15 minutes | **cooking:** 35 minutes | **serves:** 4

1 teaspoon oil

2 leeks, finely sliced

1 carrot, chopped

1 celery stalk, chopped

8 oz lean boneless, skinless chicken, finely sliced

2 tablespoons pearl barley, prepared and cooked according to package directions

3½ cups Chicken Stock (see below)

2 tablespoons chopped parsley

salt, if liked, and pepper

1 Heat the oil in a medium pan, add the leeks, carrot, and celery and fry for 3–4 minutes until beginning to soften. Add the chicken and continue to fry for 2 minutes. Add the barley and stock and bring to a boil. Reduce the heat and simmer for 20 minutes.

2 Transfer half the soup to a food processor or blender and process until smooth. Return to the pan with the parsley and season well with salt, if liked, and pepper. Heat through and serve.

nutritional values per serving | Cals **122 (513 kJ)** | Protein **15 g** | Carb **8 g** | Fat **3 g**

chicken stock

preparation: 5–10 minutes | **cooking:** about 2½ hours | **makes:** about 4 cups

cooked chicken carcass

raw giblets and trimmings

1 onion, chopped

2 carrots, chopped

1 celery stalk, chopped

1 bay leaf

a few parsley stalks, lightly crushed

1 sprig of thyme

7½ cups water

1 Chop a cooked chicken carcass into 3 or 4 pieces and place it in a large pan with the other ingredients. Bring to a boil, removing any scum from the surface. Lower the heat and simmer for 2–2½ hours. Strain and cool before refrigerating.

cauliflower and cumin soup

preparation: 10 minutes | **cooking:** 20 minutes | **serves:** 4

1 teaspoon oil

1 onion, chopped

1 garlic clove, crushed

1 teaspoon cumin seeds

1 cauliflower, cut into florets

1 large potato, chopped

generous 1¾ cups Vegetable Stock (see page 32)

generous 1¾ cups milk

2 tablespoons lowfat sour cream

2 tablespoons chopped cilantro

salt, if liked, and pepper

1 Heat the oil in a medium pan, add the onion, garlic, and cumin seeds and fry for 3–4 minutes. Add the cauliflower, potato, stock, and milk and bring to a boil. Reduce the heat and simmer for 15 minutes.

2 Transfer to a food processor or blender and process until smooth. Stir through the sour cream and cilantro and season with salt, if liked, and pepper. Heat through and serve.

tip

This is delicious served with multigrain bread, topped with melted Gruyère cheese.

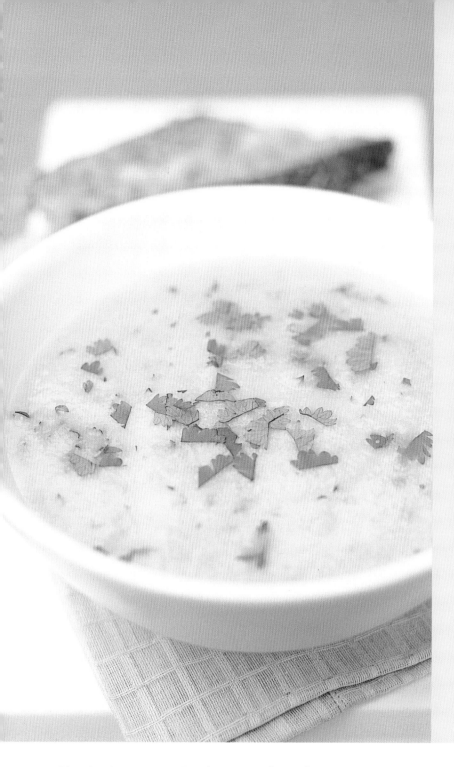

Used extensively in Middle Eastern and Indian cooking, **cumin seeds** were traditionally believed to be **good for the digestive system** and science has since backed up this claim. To release the aroma and flavor, cumin seeds should always be roasted or fried.

nutritional values per serving | Cals **152 (640 kj)** | Protein **8 g** | Carb **19 g** | Fat **6 g**

gazpacho

preparation: 15 minutes, plus chiling | **serves:** 4

1 thick slice of day-old white bread

2 tablespoons white wine vinegar

14½ oz ripe tomatoes, skinned and chopped

1 garlic clove, crushed

1¼ cups strained canned tomatoes

1¼ cups water

few drops of Tabasco sauce

1 small red bell pepper, cored, seeded, and chopped

½ cucumber, chopped

½ red onion, finely chopped

handful of basil, torn

1 tablespoon extra virgin olive oil

salt, if liked, and pepper

1 Tear the bread into pieces and soak in the vinegar. Place the tomatoes, garlic, strained tomatoes, soaked bread, and water in a food processor or blender and process until smooth. Season with salt, if liked, and pepper, and add Tabasco to taste.

2 Cover and chill in the refrigerator for at least 1 hour. Serve the soup topped with a mixture of the bell pepper, cucumber, onion, and basil, then drizzle over a little oil.

nutritional values per serving | Cals **123 (520 kj)** | Protein **5 g** | Carb **20 g** | Fat **4 g**

eggplant and chickpea pâté

preparation: 10 minutes | **cooking:** 10 minutes | **serves:** 4

1 tablespoon olive oil

1 eggplant, chopped

7 oz can chickpeas, drained and rinsed

generous ⅓ cup light cream cheese

3 scallions, finely sliced

2 tablespoons chopped mixed herbs (such as parsley, basil, and chives)

salt, if liked, and pepper

to serve

crudités

toasted whole wheat pita bread

1 Heat the oil in a nonstick pan, add the eggplant, and fry for 7–8 minutes until tender. Don't add any more oil as this is plenty. Let cool.

2 Transfer the eggplant to a food processor or blender with all the remaining ingredients and process until almost smooth but retaining a little texture. Serve the pâté with crudités and toasted pita bread.

nutritional values per serving | Cals **140 (588 kj)** | Protein **7 g** | Carb **11 g** | Fat **8 g**

herby griddled haloumi on bulgur and beet salad

preparation: 15 minutes, plus standing and cooling | **cooking:** 10 minutes | **serves:** 4

4 tablespoons chopped mixed herbs

grated rind and juice of 1 lemon

1 tablespoon toasted hazelnuts

1 tablespoon olive oil

100 g (3½ oz) haloumi or provolone cheese, cut into 8 slices

generous ¾ cup bulgur wheat

2 cooked beets, thinly sliced

2½ oz mixed salad greens

grated rind and juice of 1 orange

2 teaspoons clear honey

1 teaspoon Dijon mustard

1 Place the herbs, lemon rind and juice, hazelnuts, and oil in a food processor or blender and process until almost smooth but retaining a little texture. Pour over the cheese slices and set aside for 10 minutes.

2 Heat a griddle until hot. Lay the marinated cheese slices on the griddle and cook for 1–2 minutes on each side until beginning to brown.

3 Prepare the bulgur wheat according to the package directions. Let cool, then stir through the beets and salad greens. In a small bowl, whisk the orange rind and juice, honey, and mustard together, then drizzle over the bulgur and stir to combine. Serve the bulgur salad topped with the cheese.

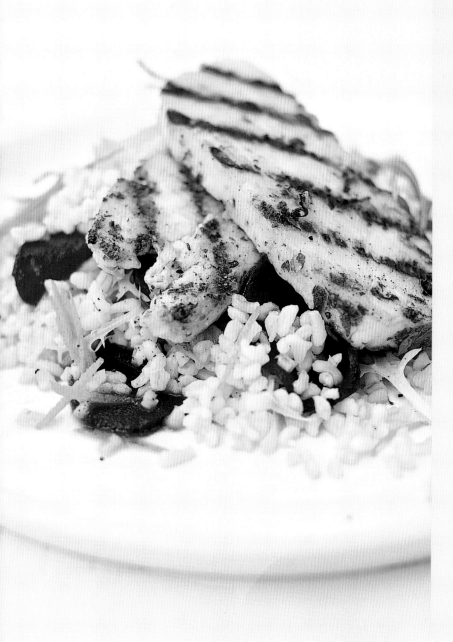

Beets are packed full of useful vitamins and minerals, including **vitamin B6, iron, calcium,** and **potassium**. It can help you fight off infection and has also been credited as a possible **anti-cancer food**.

nutritional values per serving | Cals **297 (1240 kj)** | Protein **11 g** | Carb **37 g** | Fat **13 g**

chicken and vegetable salad with a peanut dressing

preparation: 15 minutes | **serves:** 4

13 oz carrots, coarsely grated

13 oz white or savoy cabbage, shredded

2 lean boneless, skinless chicken breasts, cooked and sliced

2 cups bean sprouts

dressing

4 tablespoons peanut butter

8 tablespoons coconut milk

1 fresh red chili, finely chopped

2 tablespoons chopped cilantro

flour tortillas or pita bread, to serve

1 In a large bowl, mix all the salad ingredients together. In a small bowl, whisk all the dressing ingredients together.

2 Drizzle the dressing over the salad and toss together. Serve the salad with flour tortillas or pita bread, to make a tasty wrap or sandwich.

nutritional values per serving | Cals **277 (1157 kJ)** | Protein **25 g** | Carb **17 g** | Fat **12 g**

eggs baked with spinach and ham

preparation: 10 minutes | **cooking:** 15 minutes | **serves:** 4

6 oz baby spinach leaves

1 tablespoon water

4 oz sliced cooked ham, chopped

1 tomato, sliced into 4

4 eggs

4 tablespoons lowfat sour cream

1½ oz sharp Cheddar cheese, grated

salt, if liked, and pepper

multigrain bread, to serve

1 Place the spinach in a pan with the water and heat gently for 2–3 minutes until the spinach is wilted.

2 Divide the spinach between 4 mini ovenproof bowls or dariole molds, top with ham and a tomato slice, then crack an egg into each. Spoon a tablespoon of sour cream over each, sprinkle with Cheddar, and season with salt, if liked, and pepper.

3 Place on a cookie sheet and bake in a preheated oven, 400°F, for 10 minutes until the eggs are just set. Serve with multigrain bread to dip in the juices.

nutritional values per serving | Cals **178 (740 kJ)** | Protein **14 g** | Carb **2 g** | Fat **13 g**

blue cheese soufflés with chicory and walnut salad

preparation: 25 minutes | **cooking:** 10–12 minutes | **serves:** 4

2 tablespoons polyunsaturated margarine

⅓ cup all-purpose flour

1¼ cups milk

4 eggs, separated

3½ oz Stilton cheese, crumbled

1 teaspoon chopped thyme

oil, for oiling

4 heads of chicory, leaves separated

handful of watercress

1 tablespoon walnuts, toasted

2 tablespoons fat-free dressing

pepper

1 Melt the margarine in a medium pan, add the flour, and stir over the heat for 1 minute. Gradually add the milk, whisking constantly, and cook until thickened.

2 Remove from the heat and beat in the egg yolks, one at a time. Stir in the Stilton and thyme and season well with pepper. In a large, clean bowl, whisk the egg whites until they form firm peaks. Gradually fold them into the cheese mixture.

3 Transfer to 4 lightly oiled ramekins and bake in a preheated oven, 375°F, for 10–12 minutes until risen and golden. Toss the remaining ingredients together and serve with the soufflés.

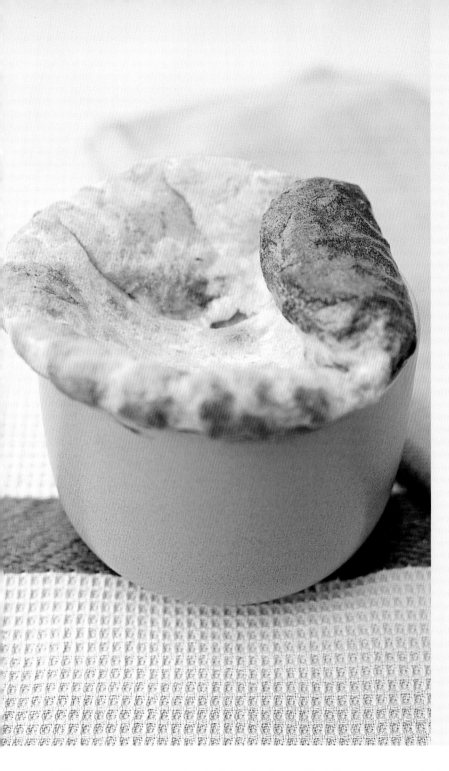

Walnuts are a great source of **potassium** and **vitamin E,** as well as being **rich in beneficial omega-3 and omega-6 oils**. Store them in the refrigerator or in a cool, dry place in an airtight container to keep fresh.

nutritional values per serving | Cals **360 (1505 kj) |** Protein **18 g |** Carb **16 g |** Fat **26 g**

new potato, watercress, and bacon salad

preparation: 10 minutes, plus standing | **cooking:** 20 minutes | **serves:** 4

1 lb 13 oz baby new potatoes, scrubbed

4 lean Canadian bacon slices, chopped

2 tablespoons olive oil

1 teaspoon Dijon mustard

juice of 1 lemon

1 teaspoon clear honey

5 oz watercress, coarsely chopped

2 heads of red chicory or radicchio, cut into bite-size pieces

pepper

1 Cook the potatoes in a pan of boiling water for 12–15 minutes until tender. Drain and tip into a serving bowl.

2 Cook the bacon in a dry, nonstick pan for 3–4 minutes until crisp. Add the oil, mustard, lemon juice, and honey and stir well. Tip into the bowl with the potatoes, mix together, and set aside for 30 minutes. Stir through the remaining ingredients and season well with pepper. Serve.

nutritional values per serving | Cals **260 (1096 kj)** | Protein **10 g** | Carb **39 g** | Fat **9 g**

turkey and avocado salad with toasted seeds

preparation: 10 minutes | **serves:** 4

14½ oz cooked turkey, sliced

1 large avocado, sliced

2 red apples, cored and sliced

1 punnet of mustard cress

4 oz mixed salad greens

2 oz toasted mixed seeds (such as pumpkin and sunflower)

dressing

3 tablespoons apple juice

3 tablespoons lowfat plain yogurt

1 teaspoon clear honey

1 teaspoon whole grain mustard

whole grain rye bread, to serve

1 In a large bowl, toss all the salad ingredients together. In a separate bowl, whisk all the dressing ingredients together.

2 Pour the dressing over the salad, mix together well, and serve with slices of whole grain rye bread.

nutritional values per serving | Cals **372 (1557 kJ)** | Protein **39 g** | Carb **15 g** | Fat **18 g**

bulgur wheat salad with fennel, orange, and spinach

preparation: 10 minutes, plus cooling | **cooking:** 15 minutes | **serves:** 4

generous ¾ cup bulgur wheat

2 tablespoons olive oil

2 fennel bulbs, finely sliced

6 oz baby spinach leaves

3 oranges, segmented

2 tablespoons pumpkin seeds, toasted

dressing

4 tablespoons plain yogurt

2 tablespoons chopped cilantro

½ small cucumber, finely chopped

salt, if liked, and pepper

1 Prepare the bulgur wheat according to the package directions. Set aside to cool. Heat half the oil in a skillet, add the fennel, and fry for 8–10 minutes until tender and browned. Add the spinach to the pan and stir through until just wilted.

2 Toss through the bulgur wheat, then the orange segments and pumpkin seeds. Mix all the dressing ingredients together with the remaining oil, stir through the salad, and serve.

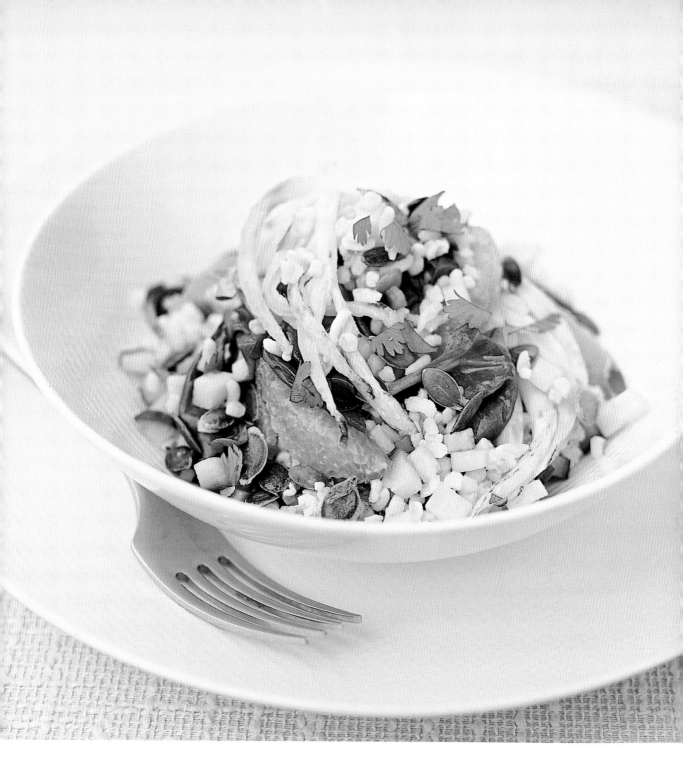

nutritional values per serving | Cals **296 (1237 kj)** | Protein **10 g** | Carb **44 g** | Fat **9 g**

lowfat chicken Caesar salad

preparation: 15 minutes | **cooking:** 10 minutes | **serves:** 4

4 small chicken breasts

1 tablespoon olive oil

2 romaine lettuces, chopped

½ cucumber, sliced

croutons

4 slices of whole grain bread

1 garlic clove, halved

dressing

3 tablespoons lowfat sour cream

1 anchovy fillet, chopped

grated rind and juice of ½ lemon

2 tablespoons freshly grated Parmesan cheese

salt, if liked, and pepper

1 Brush the chicken breasts with a little of the oil and season well with pepper. Heat a griddle until hot, lay on the chicken breasts, and cook for 3–4 minutes on each side until cooked through. Slice each chicken breast.

2 Divide the lettuce and cucumber between 4 serving plates and top each with a sliced chicken breast.

3 To make the croutons, drizzle the remaining oil over the bread and broil until toasted on each side. Rub all over with the cut sides of the garlic, cut the toast into cubes, and add to the salad.

4 Blend all the dressing ingredients together and drizzle over the salad. Serve.

nutritional values per serving | Cals **279 (1170 kj)** | Protein **28 g** | Carb **18 g** | Fat **11 g**

tortilla pizza

preparation: 10 minutes | **cooking:** 10 minutes | **serves:** 4

4 medium flour tortillas

4 tomatoes, thinly sliced

2 pears, peeled, cored, and thinly sliced

3½ oz Gorgonzola cheese, or other blue cheese, crumbled

4 tablespoons lowfat sour cream

2½ oz arugula

pepper

1 Place the tortillas on a cookie sheet (or two if needed). Layer the tomatoes, pears, and Gorgonzola over the tortillas, spoon over the sour cream, and season with pepper.

2 Cook in a preheated oven, 425°F, for 10 minutes until the cheese is bubbling. Scatter over the arugula and serve.

nutritional values per serving | Cals **274 (1150 kj)** | Protein **10 g** | Carb **35 g** | Fat **11 g**

homemade hummus with roasted vegetables in tortillas

preparation: 10 minutes | **cooking:** 45 minutes | **serves:** 4

13 oz can chickpeas, drained and rinsed

1 garlic clove

2 tablespoons strained plain yogurt

juice of 1 lemon

pinch of paprika

1 eggplant, cut into thin sticks

1 red bell pepper, cored, seeded, and sliced

2 zucchini, sliced

2 carrots, cut into thin sticks

1 red onion, sliced

1 tablespoon olive oil

1 teaspoon chopped thyme

8 small flour tortillas

1 Place the chickpeas, garlic, yogurt, lemon juice, and paprika in a food processor or blender and process until smooth. Tip into a bowl, cover, and set aside.

2 Place the vegetables in a roasting tin, drizzle over the oil, and sprinkle over the thyme. Cook in a preheated oven, 400°F, for 45 minutes until tender and beginning to char.

3 Meanwhile, warm the tortillas according to the package directions, then fill with the roasted vegetables and hummus and serve.

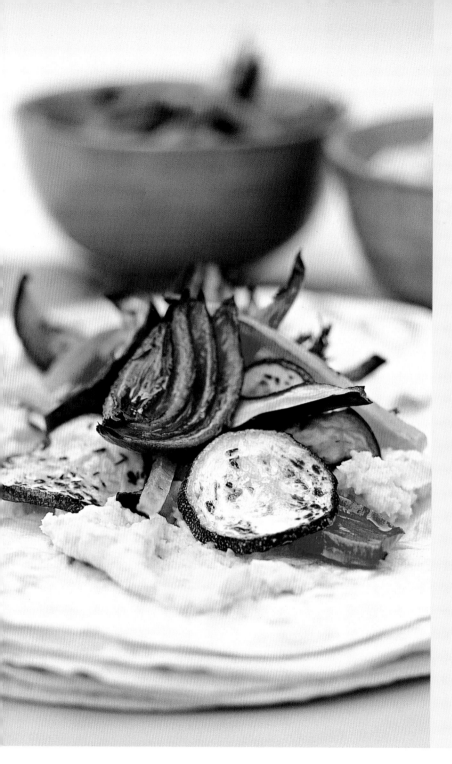

High in fiber and **protein, chickpeas,** along with lentils and other legumes, are particularly beneficial to a vegetarian diet. However, as the fiber they contain can also **help reduce cholesterol,** we should all be eating more of them.

nutritional values per serving | Cals **422 (1783 kj)** | Protein **16 g** | Carb **74 g** | Fat **9 g**

poached eggs with lentils and arugula

preparation: 10 minutes | **cooking:** 45 minutes | **serves:** 4

1¼ cups Puy lentils

generous 1¾ cups Vegetable Stock (see page 32)

1 teaspoon olive oil

4 scallions, finely sliced

3 tomatoes, chopped

4 oz arugula

4 eggs

salt, if liked, and pepper

1 Place the lentils and stock in a medium pan and bring to a boil. Reduce the heat and simmer for about 40 minutes until tender. Drain off any excess liquid.

2 Heat the oil in a skillet, add the scallions and tomatoes and fry for 2 minutes. Stir through the lentils and arugula and season with salt, if liked, and pepper.

3 Bring a large pan of lightly salted water to a boil, then reduce to a very gentle simmer and crack in one of the eggs. Swirl the water very gently to wrap the white around the yolk and cook for 3 minutes. Remove the egg from the pan and repeat with the remaining eggs. Serve on top of the lentils and arugula.

nutritional values per serving | Cals **304 (1284 kj)** | Protein **24 g** | Carb **33 g** | Fat **10 g**

creamy mushroom medley on toast

preparation: 10 minutes | **cooking:** 10 minutes | **serves:** 4

1 tablespoon olive oil

1 garlic clove, crushed (optional)

1½ lb mixed mushrooms (such as portobello, oyster, and cèpe), trimmed and sliced

1 tablespoon whole grain mustard

2 tablespoons lowfat sour cream

2 tablespoons chopped parsley

4 thick slices of whole wheat or whole grain toast

1 Heat the oil in a large skillet, add the garlic, if liked, and fry for 1 minute. Add the mushrooms and sauté for 5–6 minutes until tender.

2 Stir in the mustard, sour cream, and parsley and bring to a boil. Remove from the heat and serve on the whole wheat or whole grain toast.

nutritional values per serving | Cals **206 (869 kJ)** | Protein **9 g** | Carb **27 g** | Fat **7 g**

spinach, lima bean, and ricotta frittata

preparation: 10 minutes | **cooking:** 10 minutes | **serves:** 2

1 teaspoon olive oil

1 onion, sliced

13 oz can lima beans, drained and rinsed

7 oz baby spinach leaves

4 eggs, beaten

scant ¼ cup ricotta cheese

salt, if liked, and pepper

tomato and onion salad, to serve

1 Heat the oil in a medium skillet, add the onion, and fry for 3–4 minutes until softened. Add the lima beans and spinach and heat gently for 2–3 minutes until the spinach has wilted.

2 Pour over the eggs, then spoon over the ricotta and season with salt, if liked, and pepper. Cook until almost set, then place under a hot broiler and cook for 1–2 minutes until golden and set. Serve with a tomato and onion salad.

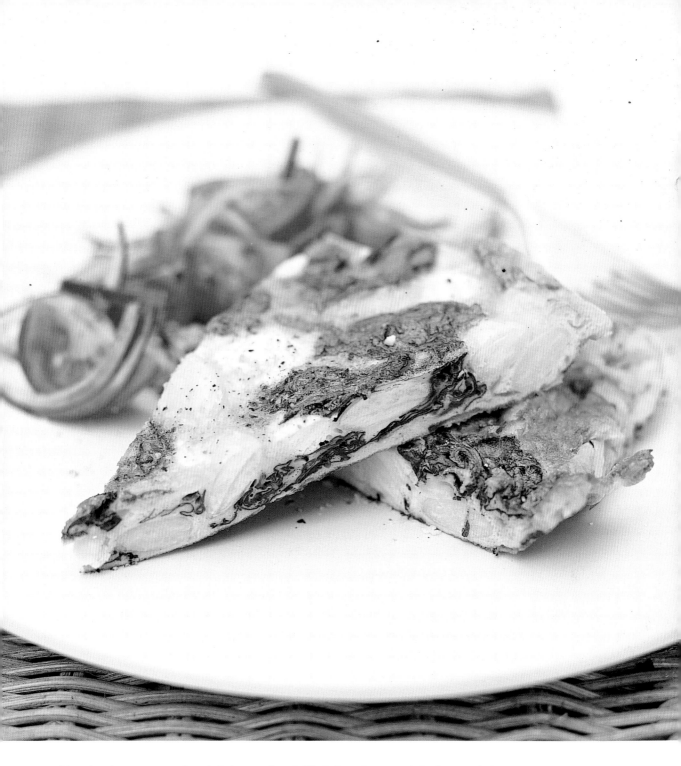

nutritional values per serving | Cals **417 (1748 kj)** | Protein **32 g** | Carb **34 g** | Fat **18 g**

lentil and corn fritters with salsa

preparation: 10 minutes | **cooking:** 10 minutes | **makes:** 16–20 fritters (serves 4)

½ cup small green lentils

3 eggs, beaten

⅔ cup milk

1 cup self-rising flour

handful of cilantro, chopped

3 scallions, sliced

1 fresh red chili, chopped

11 oz can corn kernels, drained

2 tablespoons olive oil

scant 1 cup Tomato Salsa (see right)

1 Prepare and cook the lentils according to the package directions, then drain and set aside to cool. In a bowl, beat the eggs, milk, and flour together and stir in the drained lentils, cilantro, scallions, chili, and corn.

2 Heat a little of the oil in a nonstick skillet and add tablespoons of the mixture to the pan. Fry for 1–2 minutes on each side until golden, then continue with the remaining mixture. Serve with the Tomato Salsa. The fritters are also great served with a little lowfat sour cream and smoked salmon.

tip

If you prefer, you could use the same quantity of prepared and cooked split peas instead of the lentils.

tomato salsa

preparation: 10 minutes, plus standing | **serves:** 4

1 lb cherry tomatoes, chopped

1 red onion, finely chopped

grated rind and juice of 1 lime

1 fresh green chili, finely chopped

handful of cilantro, chopped

salt, if liked, and pepper

1 Simply combine all the ingredients in a large, non-metallic bowl, cover, and allow the flavors to develop for about 30 minutes.

nutritional values per serving | Cals **438 (1852 kj)** | Protein **19 g** | Carb **66 g** | Fat **13 g**

sautéed chicken livers with wilted baby spinach

preparation: 5 minutes | **cooking:** 10 minutes | **serves:** 4

1 tablespoon olive oil

1 garlic clove, crushed

1 teaspoon chopped thyme

14½ oz chicken livers

6 oz baby spinach leaves

1 tablespoon balsamic vinegar

pepper

4 thick slices of whole wheat or whole grain bread, toasted, to serve

1 Heat the oil in a medium skillet, add the garlic, and fry for 1 minute. Add the thyme and chicken livers to the pan and fry for 2–3 minutes.

2 Stir in the spinach and balsamic vinegar and cook for 1–2 minutes until the spinach has wilted. Season with pepper and serve on whole wheat or whole grain toast.

nutritional values per serving | Cals **318 (1340 kj)** | Protein **28 g** | Carb **27 g** | Fat **12 g**

DELECTABLE DINNERS

This range of recipes shows just how flexible following a low-GI eating plan really is. Whether it's quick after-work meals or something a bit special, look no farther.

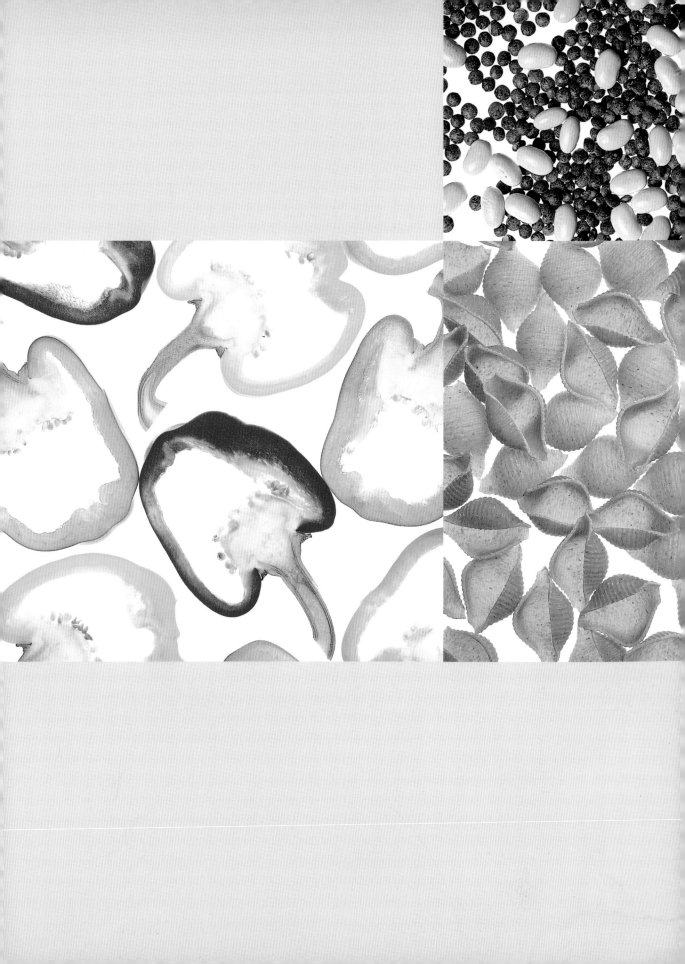

lamb with braised lentils

preparation: 15 minutes | **cooking:** 35 minutes | **serves:** 4

4 lean lamb steaks

grated rind and juice of 1 lemon

1 tablespoon chopped rosemary

1 garlic clove, crushed

2 lean smoked Canadian bacon slices, chopped

2 onions, sliced

1 carrot, finely chopped

1 celery stalk, finely chopped

1¼ cups green or Puy lentils

generous 1¾ cups Vegetable Stock (see page 32)

1 Rub the lamb steaks with the lemon rind, rosemary, and garlic, and squeeze over the lemon juice. Heat a large, nonstick skillet until hot, add the lamb steaks, and fry for 1 minute on each side.

2 Remove the lamb from the pan. Add the bacon, onions, carrot, and celery to the pan and fry for 2–3 minutes until beginning to soften. Add the lentils and stock, then return the lamb to the pan and bring to a boil. Reduce the heat and simmer gently for 30–40 minutes until the lentils are tender and most of the stock is absorbed.

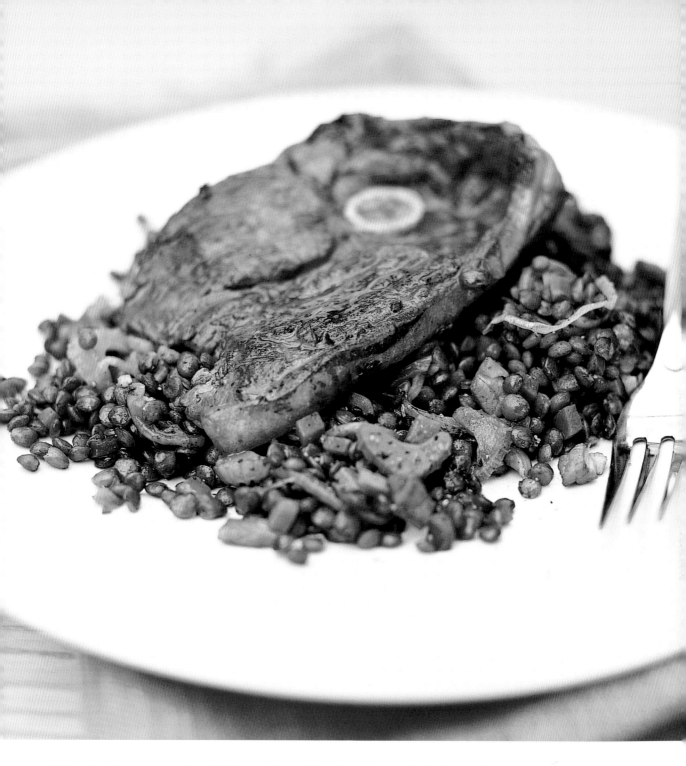

nutritional values per serving | Cals **492 (2073 kJ)** | Protein **50 g** | Carb **38 g** | Fat **17 g**

braised lamb with fruity pilaf

preparation: 10 minutes | **cooking:** about 2 hours | **serves:** 4

4 lamb shanks, about 7 oz each

12 small rosemary sprigs

4 garlic cloves, each cut into 3 slices

1 teaspoon olive oil

2 onions, cut into wedges

2½ cups lamb or beef stock

1 cup long-grain rice

12 no-soak dried apricots

4 dried figs, halved

pepper

seasonal vegetables, to serve

1 Make 3 deep incisions into each lamb shank and insert a rosemary sprig and a piece of garlic into each incision. Season well with pepper.

2 Heat the oil in a large, flameproof casserole, add the lamb shanks and onions, and fry for 4–5 minutes, turning, until browned all over. Pour over the stock and bring to a boil. Reduce the heat, cover, and simmer very gently for 1½ hours until the meat is tender.

3 Add the rice and fruit to the pan, cover, and cook for 10–12 minutes until the stock is absorbed and the rice is cooked. Serve with seasonal vegetables.

beef stock

preparation: 15 minutes | **cooking:** about 4½ hours | **makes:** about 1¼ quarts

1½ lb beef for stew, cubed

2 onions, chopped

2–3 carrots, chopped

2 celery stalks, chopped

1 bay leaf

1 bouquet garni

4–6 black peppercorns

7½ cups water

½ teaspoon salt

1 Place all the ingredients in a large pan. Slowly bring to a boil, and immediately reduce the heat to a slow simmer. Cover and simmer for 4 hours, removing any scum from the surface. Strain.

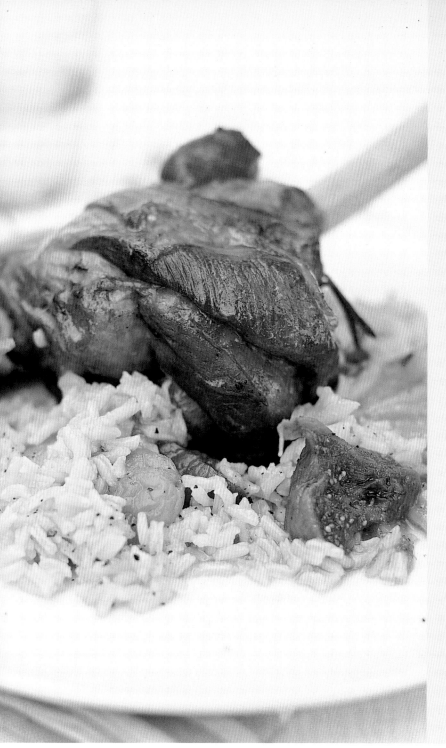

High in fiber and **vitamin C, apricots** are good for **boosting your immune system** and easing constipation. They also make a great snack.

nutritional values per serving | Cals **599 (2518 kj)** | Protein **39 g** | Carb **79 g** | Fat **15 g**

lemon grass chicken with wok-fried vegetables

preparation: 15 minutes | **cooking:** about 10 minutes | **serves:** 4

18 lemon grass stalks

8 boneless, skinless chicken thighs

1 garlic clove

2 lime leaves

2 tablespoons soy sauce

1 teaspoon sesame oil

1 red bell pepper, cored, seeded, and sliced

1 green bell pepper, cored, seeded, and sliced

12 oz sugar snap peas

2 bok choy, quartered lengthwise

1 Place 16 of the lemon grass stalks in a bowl of water and let soak for 1 hour. Chop the remaining 2 stalks.

2 Place the chicken, chopped lemon grass, garlic, lime leaves, and half the soy sauce in a food processor and process until well combined. Divide the mixture into 16 portions and mold each portion around a piece of the soaked lemon grass.

3 Place on a cookie sheet, drizzle with half the oil, and cook under a hot broiler for 4–5 minutes, turning occasionally, until golden and cooked through.

4 Heat the remaining oil in a wok or skillet, add the vegetables, and stir-fry for 2–3 minutes until just tender, then add the remaining soy sauce. Serve the stir-fried vegetables with the chicken.

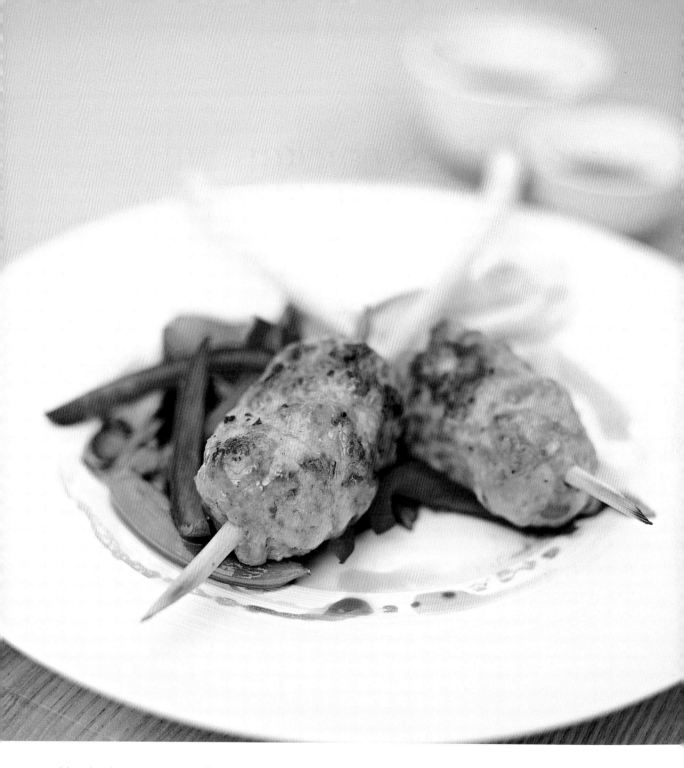

nutritional values per serving | Cals **190 (805 kj)** | Protein **25 g** | Carb **9 g** | Fat **7 g**

stuffed chicken with sautéed greens and seeds

preparation: 10 minutes | **cooking:** 30 minutes | **serves:** 4

4 large boneless, skinless chicken thighs

3 oz mozzarella cheese, cut into 4 slices

¼ cup toasted walnuts, chopped

2 tablespoons chopped parsley

8 no-soak dried apricots, chopped

2 teaspoons olive oil

2 oz pancetta, finely chopped

1 savoy cabbage, shredded

1 oz mixed seeds (such as pumpkin, sesame, and sunflower)

1 Open out the chicken thighs, then beat a little to flatten slightly. Lay a piece of mozzarella on each chicken piece. Mix the walnuts, parsley, and apricots together and divide between the chicken pieces. Roll up each chicken piece and secure with a toothpick.

2 Heat half the oil in a nonstick skillet, add the chicken, and fry for 2–3 minutes, turning, until browned all over. Place the chicken on a cookie sheet and bake in a preheated oven, 400°F, for 20 minutes until cooked through and the cheese begins to ooze.

3 Meanwhile, heat the remaining oil in a pan. Add the pancetta and fry for 2 minutes, then add the cabbage and mixed seeds and continue to fry for 5 minutes until the cabbage is tender. Serve with the chicken.

nutritional values per serving | Cals **350 (1467 kj)** | Protein **28 g** | Carb **20 g** | Fat **18 g**

baked sweet potato with griddled herb chicken

preparation: 10 minutes, plus marinating | **cooking:** about 1¼ hours | **serves:** 4

4 sweet potatoes, about 8 oz each

4 boneless, skinless chicken breasts

6 tablespoons chopped mixed herbs (such as mint, parsley, cilantro, and oregano)

1 garlic clove

1 tablespoon capers

2 teaspoons clear honey

1 tablespoon Dijon mustard

1 tablespoon olive oil

4 tablespoons light cream cheese

pepper

1 Place the potatoes on a cookie sheet and cook in a preheated oven, 400°F, for 1–1¼ hours until tender.

2 Meanwhile, cut 3 slices into the flesh of the chicken (be careful you don't cut all the way through). Place the herbs, garlic, capers, honey, mustard, and a little of the oil in a food processor or blender and process until well combined. Rub this mixture over the chicken, cover, and let stand in the refrigerator for at least 30 minutes for the flavors to develop.

3 Heat a griddle until hot, drizzle the remaining oil over the chicken, then place the chicken on the griddle and cook for 3–4 minutes on each side until beginning to char and the chicken is cooked through.

4 Cut the sweet potatoes open, spoon in some cream cheese, and season with plenty of pepper. Serve with the chicken.

nutritional values per serving | Cals **435 (1842 kj)** | Protein **34 g** | Carb **52 g** | Fat **12 g**

griddled duck with plum confit and layered potatoes

preparation: 15 minutes | **cooking:** 1 hour | **serves:** 4

14½ oz new potatoes, scrubbed
and thinly sliced

2 garlic cloves, thinly sliced

1 teaspoon chopped thyme

2 tablespoons olive oil

⅔ cup water

4 boneless duck breasts,
skinned

4 teaspoons Chinese five-spice
powder

2 large onions, sliced

1 tablespoon sugar

2 tablespoons white wine
vinegar

6 plums, halved, pitted and
sliced

pepper

steamed green vegetables,
to serve

1 Layer the potatoes, garlic, and thyme in a shallow, ovenproof dish. Mix half the oil and the water together, pour over the potatoes, and season well with pepper. Cover with foil and cook in a preheated oven, 350°F, for 1 hour until the potatoes are tender, removing the foil halfway through cooking.

2 Meanwhile, rub the skin of the duck with the five-spice powder, place on a hot griddle or in a hot skillet and fry for 3–4 minutes on each side, draining off any excess fat.

3 Heat the remaining oil in a small pan, add the onions and sugar, and fry for 10 minutes until caramelized. Add the vinegar and plums, season with pepper, and continue to cook for an additional 10 minutes.

4 Slice the duck and serve with the potatoes and plum confit, and plenty of green vegetables.

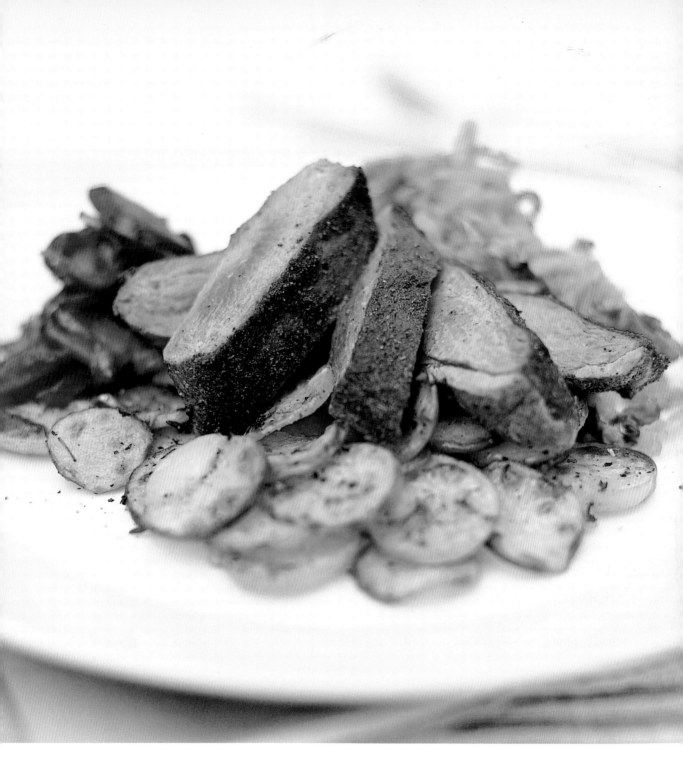

nutritional values per serving | Cals **375 (1575 kj)** | Protein **30 g** | Carb **39 g** | Fat **12 g**

Bolognese-filled pasta shells with cheeses

preparation: 15 minutes | **cooking:** 35 minutes | **serves:** 4

1 teaspoon olive oil

1 onion, chopped

1 celery stalk, chopped

1 carrot, chopped

7 oz mushrooms, sliced

14½ oz turkey mince

1¼ cups strained canned tomatoes

2 tablespoons chopped parsley

16 large whole wheat pasta shells, cooked according to package directions

generous ⅓ cup ricotta cheese

2 tablespoons freshly grated Parmesan cheese

pepper

salad, to serve

1 Heat the oil in a large skillet, add the onion, celery, carrot, and mushrooms, and fry for 3–4 minutes until softened.

2 Add the turkey mince and continue to fry, stirring to break up, for 5 minutes until browned. Pour the strained tomatoes over the mince and bring to a boil. Reduce the heat and simmer for 20 minutes. Stir through the parsley and season well with pepper.

3 Place the pasta shells in a large, ovenproof dish and divide the Bolognese mixture between them. Spoon a little ricotta on top of each, then sprinkle over the Parmesan. Bake in a preheated oven, 400°F, for 10 minutes until golden and bubbling. Serve with a salad.

nutritional values per serving | Cals **515 (2189 kj)** | Protein **43 g** | Carb **68 g** | Fat **10 g**

gourmet "Greek" burgers

preparation: 10 minutes | **cooking:** about 10 minutes | **serves:** 4

14½ oz steak mince

1 tablespoon sun-dried tomato paste

2 teaspoons chopped oregano

2 oz feta cheese, crumbled

a little beaten egg

4 whole wheat rolls, toasted

1 red onion, sliced

1 Boston lettuce, leaves separated

pepper

1 In a large bowl, mix the steak mince, tomato paste, oregano, and feta together. Season well with pepper, and stir through enough beaten egg to bind. Form the mixture into 4 burgers.

2 Place the burgers under a hot broiler and cook for 4–5 minutes on each side until browned and cooked through. Make up the burgers in the rolls, with the onion and lettuce, and serve with a napkin.

nutritional values per serving | Cals **324 (1364 kj)** | Protein **30 g** | Carb **27 g** | Fat **11 g**

spice-crusted beef tenderloin with cannellini bean mash

preparation: 10 minutes | **cooking:** 15 minutes | **serves:** 4

1 teaspoon coriander seeds

1 teaspoon cumin seeds

1 teaspoon mixed peppercorns

4 tenderloin steaks, about 4 oz each

1 teaspoon olive oil

2 x 13 oz cans cannellini beans, drained and rinsed

scant ¾ cup Vegetable Stock (see page 32)

2 tablespoons lowfat sour cream

2 tablespoons chopped cilantro

1 Place the spices in a dry skillet and fry for 1 minute, then transfer to a mortar and coarsely crush with a pestle.

2 Press the steak into the spices to cover all over. Heat the oil in the pan, add the steaks, and cook for 3 minutes on each side, or until cooked to your liking.

3 Meanwhile, place the cannellini beans and stock in a pan and bring to a boil. Reduce the heat and simmer for 10 minutes, then drain. Very lightly mash the beans together with the remaining ingredients and serve with the steak.

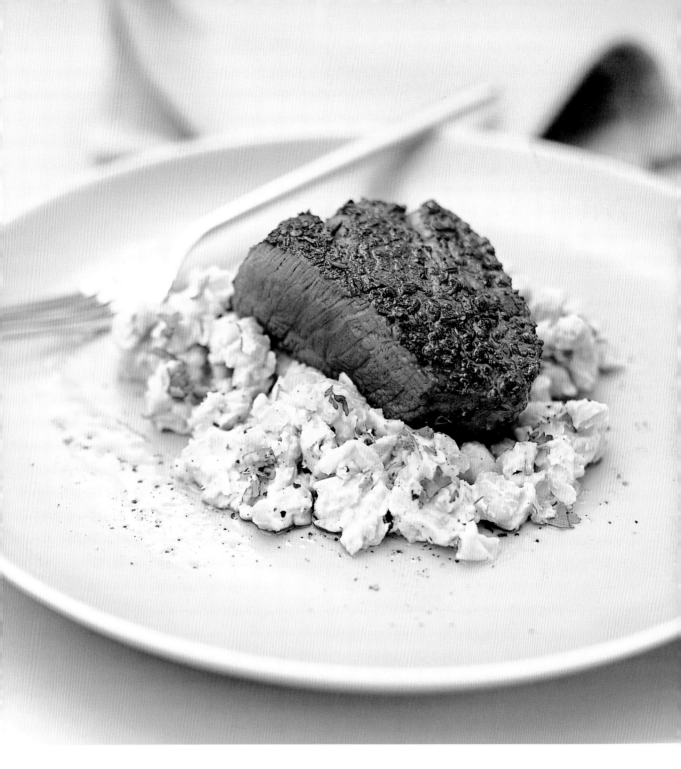

nutritional values per serving ❘ Cals **349 (1473 kJ)** ❘ Protein **37 g** ❘ Carb **27 g** ❘ Fat **11 g**

sticky pork steaks with pearl barley salad

preparation: 15 minutes, plus marinating | **cooking:** 20–25 minutes | **serves:** 4

4 lean pork steaks, about 5 oz each

2 tablespoons tomato ketchup

1 tablespoon clear honey

1 teaspoon fennel seeds

1 garlic clove, crushed

2 teaspoons Worcestershire sauce

grated rind and juice of 1 orange

1 cup pearl barley, prepared and cooked according to package directions

seeds of 1 pomegranate

4 scallions, sliced

2 tablespoons chopped mint

7 oz cherry tomatoes, quartered

1 tablespoon olive oil

1 Place the pork steaks in an ovenproof dish. Mix the ketchup, honey, fennel seeds, garlic, Worcestershire sauce, and orange rind together and pour over the steaks. Turn to coat in the sauce, then cover and let stand in the refrigerator for 30 minutes.

2 Drain the pearl barley, then toss through the pomegranate seeds, scallions, mint, tomatoes, orange juice, and oil. Cover and set aside.

3 Place the pork in a preheated oven, 425°F, and cook for 20–25 minutes until cooked and the sauce is sticky. Serve with the salad, pouring over any excess sauce.

nutritional values per serving | Cals **476 (2010 kj)** | Protein **36 g** | Carb **54 g** | Fat **15 g**

pan-fried pork with celery root and potato cakes

preparation: 20 minutes | **cooking:** 15 minutes | **serves:** 4

1 tablespoon olive oil

14½ oz pork tenderloin, cut into ½-inch slices

2 tablespoons dry white wine

2 teaspoons chopped sage

1 tablespoon whole grain mustard

3 tablespoons lowfat sour cream

1 head of celery root, about 10 oz, peeled, grated, and squeezed, to remove excess liquid

10 oz new potatoes, scrubbed, grated, and squeezed, to remove excess liquid

2 eggs, beaten

3 tablespoons all-purpose flour

3 scallions, finely sliced

pepper

steamed vegetables (such as sugar snap peas, broccoli, and carrots), to serve

1 Heat a little of the oil in a skillet. Season the pork with plenty of pepper, add to the pan, and fry for 3–4 minutes until browned all over and cooked through. Remove from the pan and keep warm.

2 Pour the wine into the pan, add the sage, and stir to deglaze the pan. Cook until reduced by half. Add the mustard and sour cream and simmer for 2 minutes. Meanwhile, in a bowl, mix the remaining ingredients, except the oil, together and form into 8 patties.

3 Heat the remaining oil in a skillet, add the potato cakes, and fry for 4–5 minutes on each side until golden, pressing down with a spatula to ensure that the mixture sticks together.

4 Place the pork on top of the potato cakes, spoon over the sauce, and serve with a selection of steamed vegetables.

nutritional values per serving | Cals **386 (1615 kJ)** | Protein **31 g** | Carb **27 g** | Fat **17 g**

chili shrimp with lime basmati

preparation: 15 minutes | **cooking:** 20 minutes | **serves:** 4

14½ oz raw jumbo shrimp, shelled

2 garlic cloves, crushed

2 fresh red chilies, finely chopped

2 tablespoons chopped cilantro

1 teaspoon sesame oil

grated rind and juice of 2 limes (reserve 2 of the lime "shells")

generous 1 cup basmati rice, rinsed

1½ cups boiling water

1 oz creamed coconut

4 tablespoons water

2 tablespoons peanuts, crushed, to garnish (optional)

1 Place the shrimp in a non-metallic bowl. Place the garlic, chilies, cilantro, oil, and half the lime rind and juice in a mortar and grind with a pestle to make a paste, or use a food processor or blender. Tip over the shrimp and stir, covering the shrimp with the paste.

2 Place the rice in a pan and pour over the 1½ cups boiling water, the lime "shells", and the remaining lime rind and juice. Bring to a boil, then reduce the heat, cover, and simmer for 12–15 minutes until the liquid is absorbed and the rice is tender and fluffy.

3 Meanwhile, heat a dry skillet until hot, then add the shrimp and fry for 2–3 minutes until they just turn pink. Add the coconut and water and bring to a boil, then reduce the heat and simmer for 1 minute. Serve the shrimp with the rice, sprinkling over the peanuts to garnish, if liked.

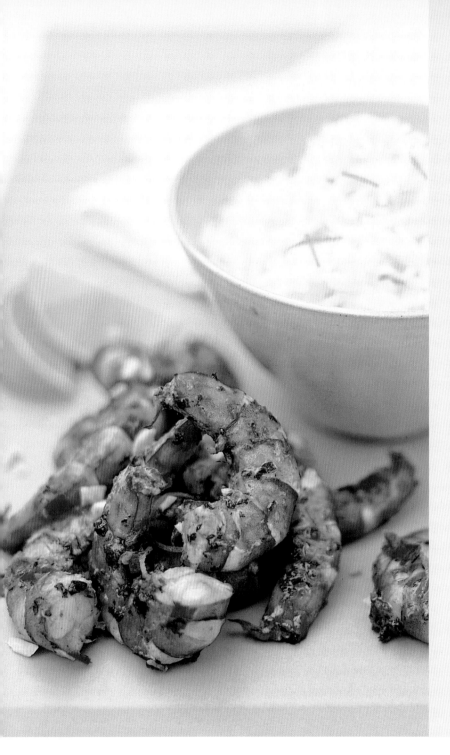

When choosing **chilies**, there's a general rule to follow: the smaller the chili, the hotter the flavor. But with their **high vitamin C content** and **antibacterial properties**, you should definitely turn up the heat.

nutritional values per serving | Cals **367 (1535 kj)** | Protein **26 g** | Carb **48 g** | Fat **7 g**

fragrant shrimp curry

preparation: 15 minutes | **cooking:** 10 minutes | **serves:** 4

6 scallions, chopped

1–2 fresh green chilies, halved

2 garlic cloves, crushed

2 teaspoons canola oil

1 teaspoon turmeric

1 teaspoon cumin seeds

1 teaspoon ground cumin

1 teaspoon mustard seeds

1 teaspoon ground coriander

5 tomatoes, chopped

2 tablespoons water

4 tablespoons heavy cream

2 oz creamed coconut, dissolved in ⅓ cup boiling water

14½ oz cooked shelled shrimp

2 tablespoons chopped cilantro

flat bread or boiled rice, to serve

1 Place the scallions, chili, and garlic in a mortar and grind with a pestle to make a paste, or use a food processor or blender.

2 Heat the oil in a pan, add the turmeric, cumin seeds, ground cumin, mustard seeds, and ground coriander and fry for 1 minute. Add the scallion paste to the pan and fry for 2–3 minutes.

3 Add the tomatoes and water to the pan and simmer for 5 minutes. Add the heavy cream and creamed coconut and simmer for an additional 2 minutes. Stir in the shrimp and cilantro, heat through, and serve with flat bread or rice.

nutritional values per serving | Cals **387 (1608 kj)** | Protein **28 g** | Carb **7 g** | Fat **27 g**

spaghetti with crab and lemon sauce

preparation: 10 minutes | **cooking:** 10 minutes | **serves:** 4

11½ oz spaghetti

1 teaspoon olive oil

bunch of scallions, sliced

2 garlic cloves, crushed

1 fresh red chili, finely sliced

10 oz cooked fresh white crab meat

grated rind and juice of 1 lemon

6 tablespoons lowfat sour cream

salt, if liked, and pepper

salad, to serve

1 Cook the spaghetti in a large pan of boiling water according to the package directions. Drain well.

2 Heat the oil in a large skillet, then add the scallions, garlic, and chili and fry for 3 minutes. Add the remaining ingredients with the cooked pasta. Season with salt, if liked, and pepper and heat through. Serve with a salad.

nutritional values per serving | Cals **459 (1944 kj)** | Protein **27 g** | Carb **68 g** | Fat **11 g**

smoked haddock and pea risotto

preparation: 10 minutes | **cooking:** 25 minutes | **serves:** 4

1 teaspoon olive oil

1 small onion, finely chopped

1¾ cups risotto rice

1 small glass dry white wine

3½ cups) Vegetable Stock, boiling (see page 32)

11½ oz smoked haddock fillet, skinned and cubed

scant 2 cups frozen peas

2 tablespoons chopped chives

3 tablespoons freshly grated Parmesan cheese, plus extra to serve (optional)

pepper

green salad, to serve

1 Heat the oil in a large, nonstick skillet, add the onion, and fry for 2–3 minutes until beginning to soften. Stir in the rice, coating it in the oil, then pour in the wine and let absorb.

2 Add the stock, a ladleful at a time, letting each amount be absorbed before adding the next. Stir constantly. Add the haddock and peas with the last ladleful of stock and cook for an additional 5 minutes until the fish flakes easily.

3 Stir in the remaining ingredients and season well with pepper. The process will take about 20 minutes. Serve with a green salad and extra grated Parmesan, if liked.

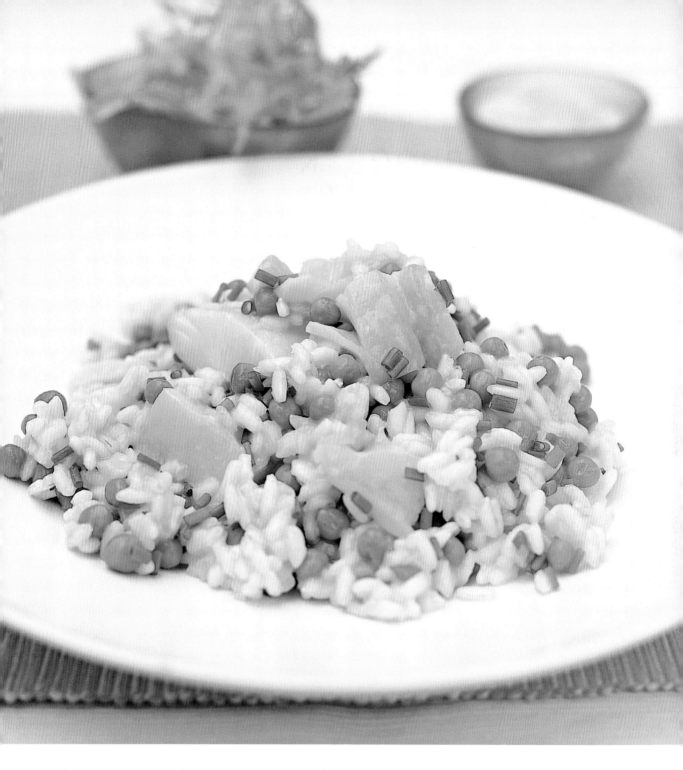

nutritional values per serving | Cals **496 (2100 kj)** | Protein **27 g** | Carb **82 g** | Fat **7 g**

baked salmon pockets

preparation: 15 minutes | **cooking:** 10–12 minutes | **serves:** 4

4 pieces of skinless salmon fillet, about 4 oz each

1 orange, cut into 8 slices

4 scallions, shredded

4 tablespoons lowfat sour cream

handful of basil leaves

salt, if liked, and pepper

to serve

boiled new potatoes

salad or steamed vegetables

1 Place each piece of salmon in the center of a 10-inch square of foil and top each with 2 orange slices. Mix the remaining ingredients together and divide between the salmon fillets.

2 Fold up each square of foil securely to enclose the salmon. Place the pockets on a cookie sheet and bake in a preheated oven, 400°F, for 10–12 minutes. Serve the salmon with new potatoes and salad or vegetables.

nutritional values per serving | Cals **287 (1196 kj)** | Protein **25 g** | Carb **5 g** | Fat **19 g**

linguine with arugula pesto and goat cheese

preparation: 10 minutes | **cooking:** 10 minutes | **serves:** 4

11½ oz linguine (or a pasta shape of your choice)

4 oz arugula

¼ cup toasted hazelnuts

1½ oz Parmesan cheese, freshly grated

3 tablespoons plain yogurt

3½ oz goat cheese, chopped

pepper

1 Cook the pasta in a large pan of boiling water according to the package directions. Drain well.

2 Meanwhile, place the arugula, hazelnuts, Parmesan, and yogurt in a food processor or blender and process until almost smooth. Toss the mixture through the pasta with the goat cheese, to warm through, season well with pepper, and serve.

nutritional values per serving | Cals **484 (2039 kj)** | Protein **22 g** | Carb **68 g** | Fat **16 g**

Asian-marinated salmon with stir-fried rice noodles

preparation: 15 minutes, plus marinating | **cooking:** about 10 minutes | **serves:** 4

4 pieces of salmon fillet, about 4 oz each

1 garlic clove, crushed

1-inch piece of fresh gingerroot, peeled and grated

2 tablespoons soy sauce

2 tablespoons rice wine vinegar

1 tablespoon sesame oil

8 oz medium rice noodles

7 oz snow peas, halved lengthwise

5 oz shiitake mushrooms, trimmed and sliced

4 scallions, sliced

2 cups bean sprouts

2 bok choy, quartered lengthwise

1 Place the salmon in a non-metallic dish. Whisk the garlic, ginger, soy sauce, vinegar, and half the oil together. Pour over the salmon, cover, and set aside in a cool place for at least 10 minutes, to allow the flavors to develop.

2 Heat a griddle or a nonstick skillet until hot, add the salmon, reserving the marinade, and cook for 2–3 minutes on each side until just cooked through. Meanwhile, cook the noodles according to the package directions, then drain.

3 Heat the remaining oil in a skillet or wok, add the snow peas, mushrooms, scallions, bean sprouts, and bok choy, and stir-fry for 3–4 minutes. Add the reserved marinade and the noodles to the pan, toss together, and heat through. Serve topped with a piece of salmon.

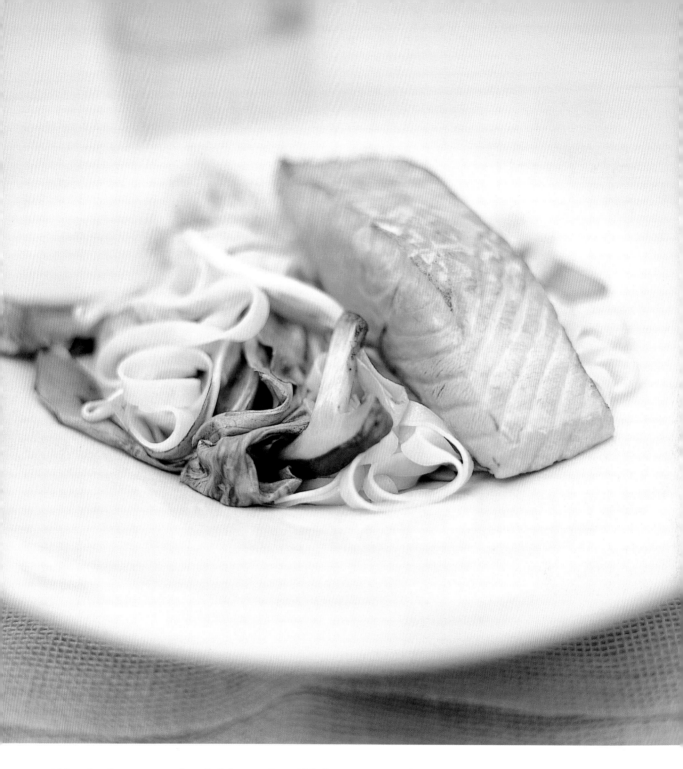

nutritional values per serving | Cals **528 (2206 kj)** | Protein **32 g** | Carb **58 g** | Fat **18 g**

tofu and tomato pasta

preparation: 10 minutes | **cooking:** 15 minutes | **serves:** 4

11½ oz whole wheat pasta
shapes

1 tablespoon olive oil

8 oz firm tofu, cut into bite-size
cubes

6 scallions, sliced

14½ oz cherry tomatoes, halved

handful of basil, torn

1 garlic clove, crushed

salt, if liked, and pepper

1 Cook the pasta in a large pan
of boiling water according to the
package directions. Drain well.

2 Meanwhile, heat the oil in a
nonstick skillet, add the tofu,
and fry for 3–4 minutes until
golden. Mix the remaining
ingredients together and toss
through the pasta with the tofu.
Season with salt, if liked, and
pepper and serve.

nutritional values per serving | Cals **378 (1600 kJ)** | Protein **18 g** | Carb **63 g** | Fat **8 g**

Moroccan vegetable stew

preparation: 20 minutes | **cooking:** 20 minutes | **serves:** 4

2 teaspoons olive oil

2 garlic cloves, sliced

2 onions, sliced

1 eggplant, chopped

1¼ lb sweet potatoes, chopped

1 teaspoon ground cumin

1 teaspoon ground coriander

½ teaspoon turmeric

2½ cups Vegetable Stock (see page 32)

7 oz green beans

13 oz can chickpeas, drained and rinsed

4 tomatoes, chopped

2 cups couscous

2 tablespoons chopped mixed herbs (such as mint, parsley, and cilantro)

grated rind and juice of 1 lemon

1 Heat the oil in a medium pan. Add the garlic and onions and fry for 2–3 minutes until beginning to soften. Add the eggplant and sweet potatoes and fry for 3–4 minutes, then add the spices and cook for 1 minute.

2 Pour the stock into the pan and bring to a boil. Reduce the heat and simmer for 10 minutes. Add the beans, chickpeas, and tomatoes and simmer for an additional 5 minutes.

3 Meanwhile, prepare the couscous according to the package directions. Mix the herbs into the couscous with the lemon rind and juice. Serve the couscous with the stew.

nutritional values per serving | Cals **529 (2234 kj)** | Protein **17 g** | Carb **106 g** | Fat **7 g**

stuffed roasted bell peppers on herby bulgur

preparation: 15 minutes | **cooking:** 30 minutes | **serves:** 4

2 red bell peppers, halved, cored, and seeded

2 yellow or orange bell peppers, halved, cored, and seeded

16 cherry tomatoes, halved

4 tablespoons cream cheese or lowfat sour cream

2 tablespoons pesto

⅔ cup bulgur wheat

grated rind and juice of 1 lemon

4 tablespoons chopped mixed herbs (such as parsley, mint, and oregano)

6 scallions, sliced

2 tablespoons pine nuts

1 Place the bell pepper halves on a cookie sheet, cut-side up. Divide the halved tomatoes between the bell peppers. Beat the cream cheese or sour cream and pesto together and spoon over the bell peppers.

2 Season the bell peppers well, then cook in a preheated oven, 400°F, for 30 minutes until tender.

3 Meanwhile, prepare the bulgur wheat according to the package directions, then stir through the lemon rind and juice, herbs, and scallions. Lightly toast the pine nuts in a dry skillet.

4 Serve the bulgur wheat with the bell peppers, sprinkled with the toasted pine nuts.

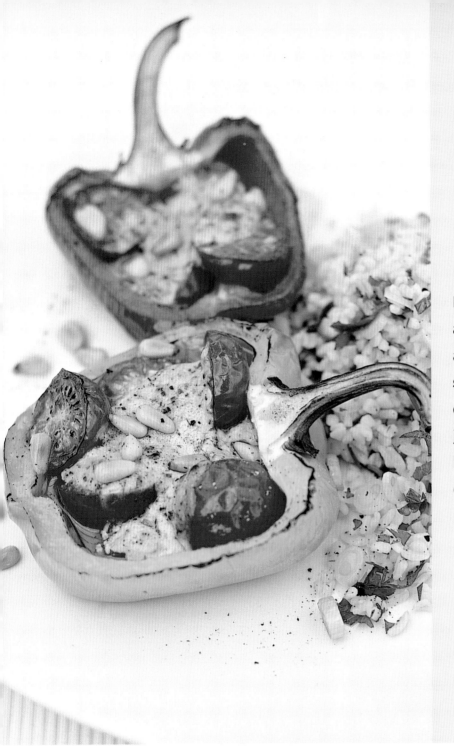

Improved blood circulation, a **strong immune system,** and **protection against strokes, heart disease, and certain cancers**; these are just some of the health benefits you could enjoy by eating **bell peppers**.

nutritional values per serving | Cals **309 (1290 kj)** | Protein **11 g** | Carb **36 g** | Fat **14 g**

SWEET TREATS

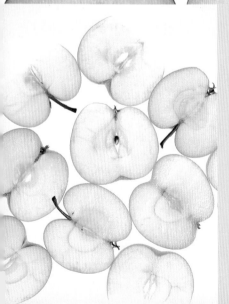

If you've got a sweet tooth, don't despair—low GI is about eating sensibly while also enjoying your food. We all need a little indulgence every now and again.

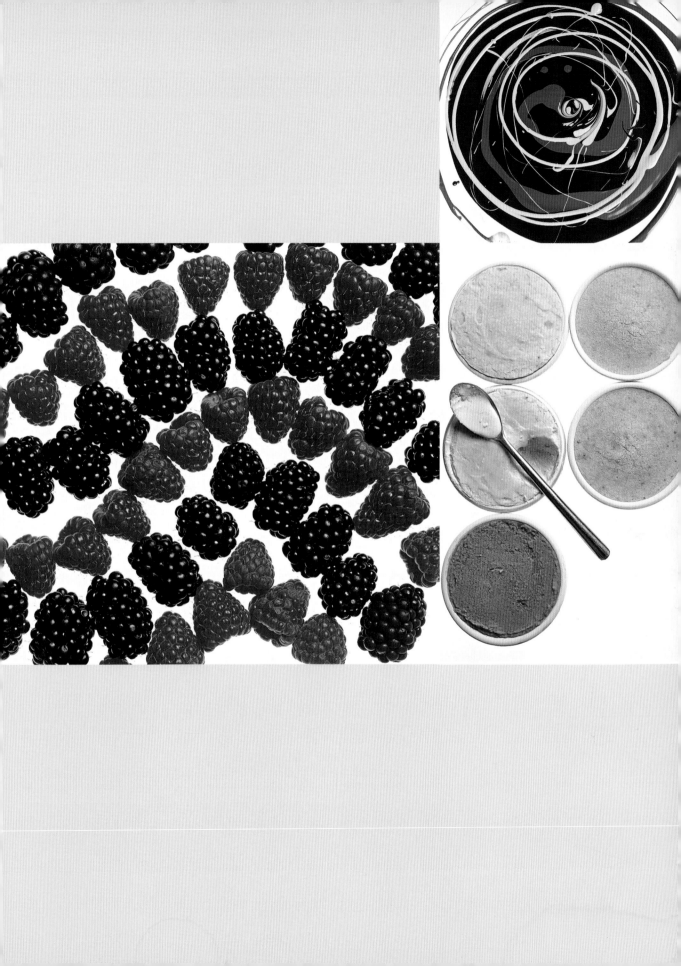

plum tatin

preparation: 15 minutes, plus cooling | **cooking:** 45 minutes | **serves:** 8

¼ cup butter or polyunsaturated margarine

¼ cup superfine sugar

1lb 3 oz plums (any variety), quartered and pitted

8 oz Short-Crust Pastry (see below)

lowfat yogurt or ice cream, to serve

1 Place the butter or margarine and sugar in an 8½-inch fixed-base cake pan over a medium heat and cook, stirring constantly, for about 5 minutes until golden.

2 Carefully arrange the plums in the pan, skin-side down. Roll out the pie dough to fit snugly over the the fruit and press down.

3 Bake in a preheated oven, 375°F, for about 40 minutes until the pastry is golden and the juices are bubbling. Let cool in the pan for 10 minutes, then invert on to a large plate and serve with a little yogurt or ice cream.

short-crust pastry

preparation: 10 minutes, plus chilling | **makes:** 11 oz

1½ cups all-purpose flour

¼ cup butter or polyunsaturated margarine, cubed and chilled

¼ cup shortening, cubed and chilled

3–4 tablespoons cold water

1 Sift the flour into a bowl, add the butter or margarine and shortening, and cut into the flour using your fingertips and a light action until the mixture resembles fine breadcrumbs. Add the cold water and bring together to form a ball. Wrap in foil and chill in the refrigerator for 30 minutes before using.

tip

You could use half whole wheat flour if you prefer, giving a pastry with a lower GI.

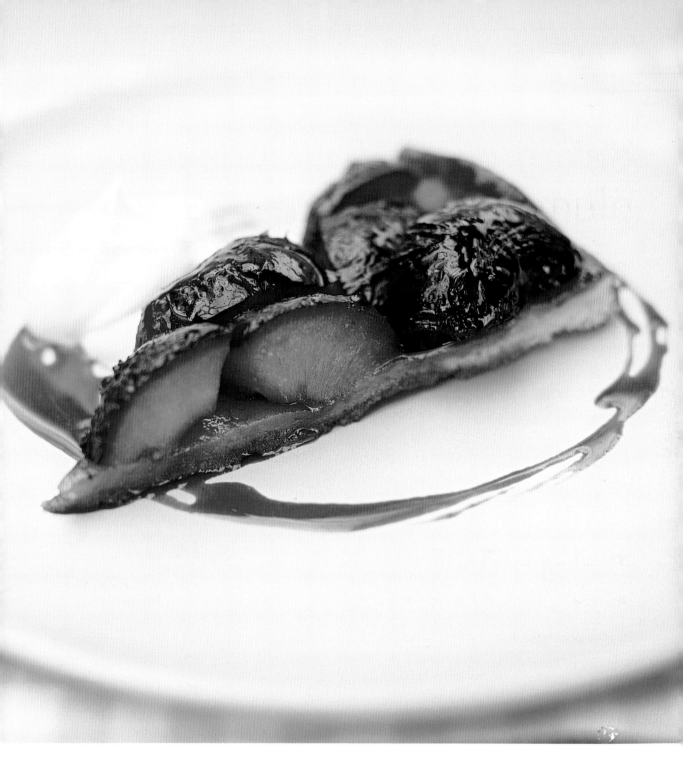

nutritional values per serving | Cals **222 (928 kj)** | Protein **2 g** | Carb **27 g** | Fat **12 g**

baked exotic fruit pockets with spiced cream

preparation: 15 minutes | **cooking:** 15 minutes | **serves:** 4

1 pineapple, prepared and cut into chunks

1 mango, peeled, pitted, and chopped

2 bananas, chopped

1⅔ cups strawberries, halved

15 oz can litchis, drained, a little juice reserved

2 pieces of preserved ginger, finely chopped

1 teaspoon allspice

4 tablespoons lowfat sour cream

1 Cut 4 x 10-inch squares of foil. Divide the fruit between the squares, add half the ginger, and drizzle over a little of the reserved litchi juice. Fold up each square of foil securely to enclose the fruit.

2 Place the pockets on a cookie sheet and cook in a preheated oven, 400°F, for 15 minutes. Mix the allspice, sour cream, and remaining ginger together and serve on the hot fruit pockets.

nutritional values per serving | Cals **230 (974 kj)** | Protein **3 g** | Carb **48 g** | Fat **4 g**

baked gooseberries with oaty topping

preparation: 10 minutes | **cooking:** 40 minutes | **serves:** 4

5 cups fresh gooseberries, prepared

2 tablespoons raw brown sugar

4 tablespoons mascarpone cheese

2 tablespoons butter or polyunsaturated margarine, melted

2 tablespoons clear honey

2 cups jumbo oats

⅓ cup chopped mixed nuts

lowfat plain yogurt, to serve

1 Place the gooseberries in an ovenproof dish, sprinkle over the sugar, and bake in a preheated oven, 400°F, for 20 minutes until they are tender and oozing juice.

2 Spoon the mascarpone over the gooseberries. Mix the remaining ingredients together and spoon over the gooseberries. Return to the oven and bake for 15 minutes. Serve with plain yogurt.

tip

If fresh gooseberries are unavailable, you can substitute the same quantity of plums or rhubarb in the recipe.

nutritional values per serving | Cals **475 (1990 kj)** | Protein **10 g** | Carb **51 g** | Fat **27 g**

cappuccino panna cotta

preparation: 10 minutes, plus cooling and chilling | **serves:** 4

1¼ cups lowfat milk

¼ cup superfine sugar

4 tablespoons heavy cream

½ teaspoon vanilla extract

2 sheets of leaf gelatin

150 g (5 oz) plain yogurt

4 tablespoons very strong cold black coffee

fresh raspberries, to serve

1 Pour the milk into a medium pan with the sugar, cream, and vanilla extract. Bring to a boil, then remove from the heat. Soak the gelatin sheets in cold water until soft.

2 Squeeze the water from the gelatin, then stir into the milk mixture until dissolved. Let cool (about 15 minutes) and then stir through the yogurt and coffee and whisk until smooth.

3 Strain, then pour the mixture into 4 dariole molds. Chill in the refrigerator for 4–6 hours until set. Remove the panna cotta from the molds by dipping the outside of each mould into a bowl of hot water for a couple of seconds, then tip on to serving plates. Serve with fresh raspberries.

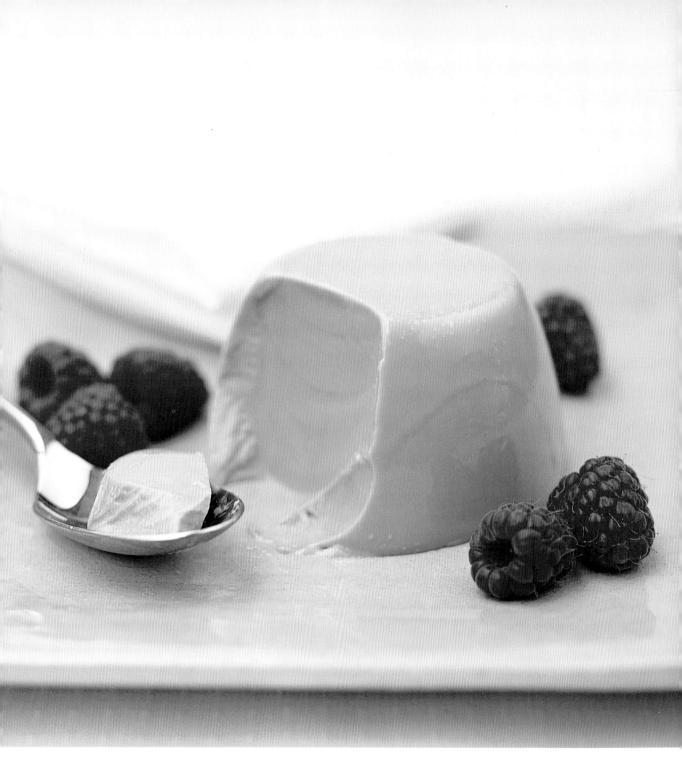

nutritional values per serving | Cals **247 (1029 kj)** | Protein **7 g** | Carb **21 g** | Fat **16 g**

instant mixed berry frozen yogurt

preparation: 5 minutes I **serves:** 4

3 cups mixed frozen summer berries (such as strawberries, raspberries, and blackberries)

1¾ oz lowfat strained plain yogurt

1 tablespoon confectioners' sugar

1 Place all the ingredients in a food processor or blender and process until smooth. Serve immediately, or store in a freezerproof container in the freezer until required.

nutritional values per serving I Cals **129 (544 kj)** I Protein **7 g** I Carb **98 g** I Fat **3 g**

grapefruit syllabub

preparation: 10 minutes | **serves:** 4

generous ¾ cup whipping cream

2 tablespoons superfine sugar

generous ¾ cup lowfat strained plain yogurt

grated rind and juice of
1 grapefruit

1 grapefruit, segmented

1 In a large bowl, whip the cream with the sugar until it forms soft peaks. Fold through the yogurt and grapefruit rind and juice.

2 Divide the grapefruit segments between 4 tall glasses, then spoon over the syllabub. Serve immediately or chill in the refrigerator until required.

nutritional values per serving | Cals **272 (1130 kj)** | Protein **4 g** | Carb **53 g** | Fat **21 g**

blackberry and apple tartlets

preparation: 15 minutes | **cooking:** 20 minutes | **serves:** 4

6 oz puff pastry, thawed if frozen

1 dessert apple, peeled, cored, and very thinly sliced

a little melted butter, for brushing

1¾ cups blackberries

2 tablespoons apricot jelly, warmed

plain yogurt to serve

1 Cut the pie dough into 4 pieces and roll each out thinly to a rectangle about 3½ x 6 inches.

2 Mark a border around the pie dough pieces, ½ inch from the edge. Lay the apple slices inside the marked square, brush with a little butter, then bake in a preheated oven, 400°F, for 15 minutes. Remove from the oven, add the blackberries, then return to the oven and continue to cook for 5 minutes.

3 Remove from the oven and brush with a little apricot jelly. Let cool, then serve the tartlets with a little plain yogurt.

tip

If blackberries are unavailable, you can substitute them for the same quantity of blueberries or raspberries.

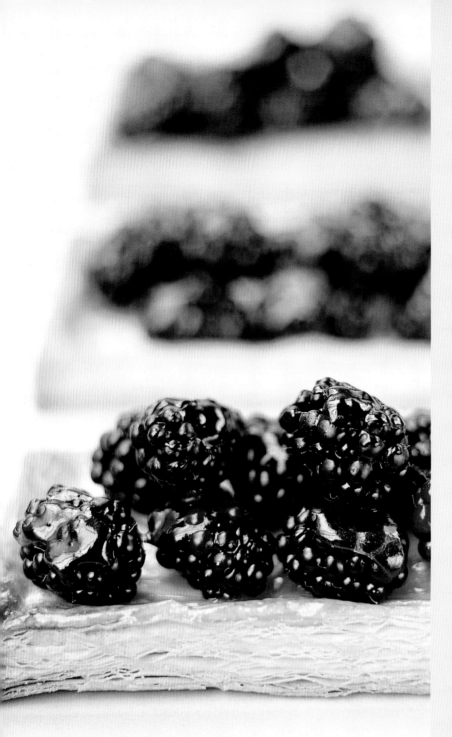

Eating **blackberries** can help **boost your immune system**. They are also good for **combating memory loss** as we get older, so tuck in now and you might never forget where you left your keys again.

nutritional values per serving | Cals **213 (890 kj)** | Protein **3 g** | Carb **28 g** | Fat **11 g**

raspberry and passion fruit fool

preparation: 10 minutes, plus overnight chilling | **serves:** 4

generous ¾ cup light evaporated milk, chilled overnight

1 tablespoon superfine sugar

3 cups raspberries

flesh of 2 passion fruit

1 In a large bowl, whip the evaporated milk and sugar together until the mixture is thick and fluffy.

2 Process half the raspberries in a food processor or blender until smooth, then stir into the whipped evaporated milk with the whole raspberries and the passion fruit. Spoon into serving dishes and serve.

nutritional values per serving | Cals **98 (414 kj)** | Protein **6 g** | Carb **14 g** | Fat **2 g**

banana and chocolate microwave sponge pudding

preparation: 10 minutes I **cooking:** 5 minutes I **serves:** 4

scant ½ cup butter or polyunsaturated margarine, plus extra for greasing

⅔ cup self-rising flour, plus extra for dusting

generous ⅓ cup superfine sugar

2 eggs

few drops of vanilla extract

⅓ cup semisweet chocolate drops

2 bananas, sliced

1 In a large bowl, beat the butter or margarine, flour, sugar, eggs, and vanilla extract together until smooth, then fold in the chocolate drops.

2 Lightly grease and flour a 2½-cup ovenproof bowl, layer in the banana, then pour over the sponge batter.

3 Cover with plastic wrap, then cook in the microwave on high for 4–5 minutes. Remove the plastic wrap immediately and let cool in the dish for 5 minutes before turning out on to a serving plate.

nutritional values per serving I Cals **494 (2069 kj)** I Protein **7 g** I Carb **58 g** I Fat **28 g**

fruity bread and butter pudding

preparation: 15 minutes, plus standing | **cooking:** about 30 minutes | **serves:** 4

2 tablespoons butter

4 thick slices of whole wheat or whole grain bread, each cut into 4 triangles

¼ cup no-soak dried apricots, chopped

4 dried figs, chopped

generous ¼ cup golden raisins

3 eggs, beaten

1¼ cups milk

generous ⅓ cup light cream

pinch of nutmeg

1 Butter the bread slices and lightly butter an ovenproof dish or bowl. Place a layer of bread in the bottom of the dish or bowl and sprinkle over some of the fruit. Repeat until all the bread and fruit is used up.

tip

For a change, you could use a mixture of fresh fruit to suit your taste, or use whatever you have to hand.

2 In a separate bowl, whisk the remaining ingredients together and pour into the dish or bowl, aiming to soak all the bread. Let stand for 30 minutes until all the liquid is soaked up, then bake in a preheated oven, 400°F, for about 30 minutes until golden and risen.

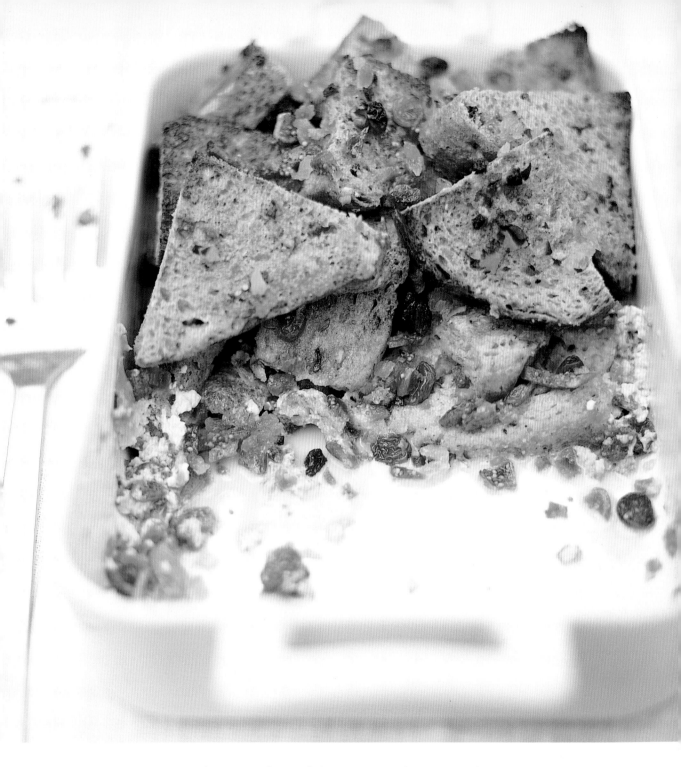

nutritional values per serving | Cals **419 (1766 kj)** | Protein **15 g** | Carb **54 g** | Fat **18 g**

simple lemon and lime cheesecake

preparation: 10 minutes | **serves:** 4

6 oaty cookies, coarsely crushed

1¼ cups vanilla or plain yogurt

generous ¾ cup light cream cheese

grated rind and juice of 1 lime

grated rind and juice of 1 lemon

2 tablespoons superfine sugar

fresh fruit, chopped, to serve

1 Divide the cookies between 4 serving dishes. Beat the remaining ingredients together and spoon on to the cookies. Serve immediately with some fresh fruit of your choice.

nutritional values per serving | Cals **287 (1208 kj)** | Protein **10 g** | Carb **37 g** | Fat **12 g**

rich chocolate mousse

preparation: 15 minutes, plus chilling | **cooking:** 2–5 minutes | **serves:** 4

5 oz semisweet chocolate

2 large eggs, separated

4 tablespoons heavy cream, whipped to form soft peaks

2 tablespoons superfine sugar

to serve

fresh fruit, chopped

plain yogurt or cream

1 Place the chocolate in a heatproof bowl and set over a pan of barely simmering water until melted. Alternatively, you can melt the chocolate in the microwave on high for 1–2 minutes.

2 Remove from the heat and let cool for a couple of minutes, then beat in the egg yolks and cream. In a clean bowl, whisk the egg whites until they form soft peaks, add the sugar, and continue to whisk until stiff peaks are formed.

3 Gently fold into the chocolate mixture, then spoon into 4 tall glasses or ramekins. Chill in the refrigerator for at least 2 hours. Serve with some fresh fruit and a spoonful of plain yogurt or cream.

nutritional values per serving | Cals **398 (1660 kj)** | Protein **6 g** | Carb **32 g** | Fat **29 g**

BAKING

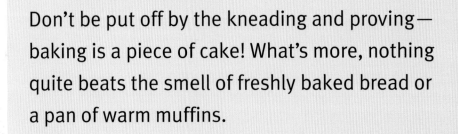

Don't be put off by the kneading and proving—
baking is a piece of cake! What's more, nothing
quite beats the smell of freshly baked bread or
a pan of warm muffins.

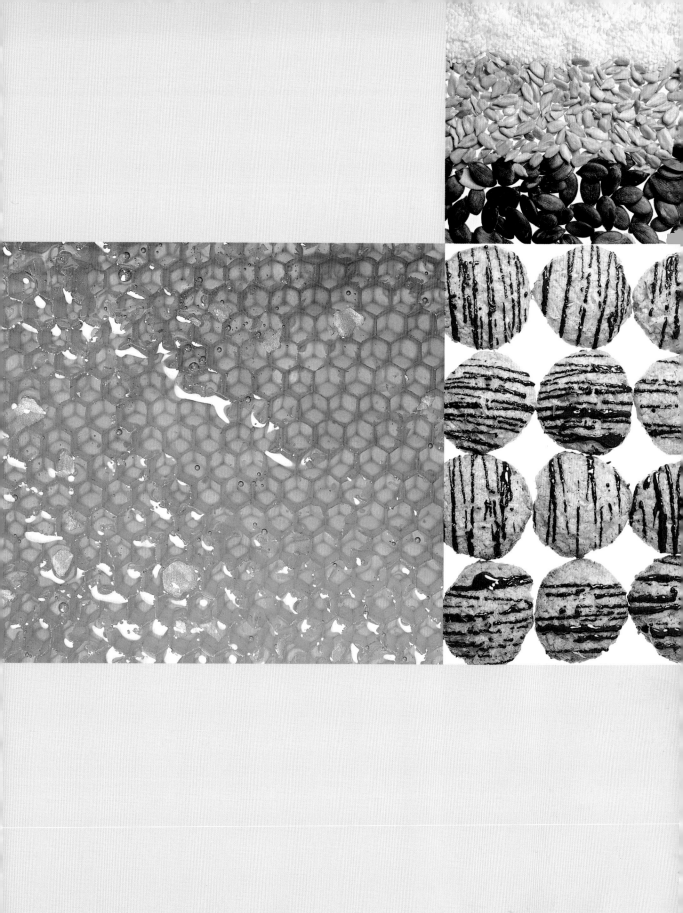

apple and apricot muffins

preparation: 20 minutes | **cooking:** 15–20 minutes | **makes:** 12

⅔ cup all-purpose whole wheat flour

1 cup all-purpose flour

1 teaspoon baking powder

1 teaspoon baking soda

2 tablespoons superfine sugar

generous ½ cup no-soak dried apricots, chopped

½ teaspoon ground cinnamon

2 red dessert apples, peeled, cored, and chopped

1 egg, beaten

¼ cup polyunsaturated margarine, melted

generous ¾ cup skim milk

1 Place 12 large muffin paper liners in a muffin pan. Sift the flours, baking powder, and baking soda together into a large bowl, tipping any bran in the strainer back into the bowl. Stir in the sugar, apricots, cinnamon, and apples.

2 In a separate bowl, whisk the remaining ingredients together, then gently stir into the flour mixture, making sure you don't beat too much as this will spoil the end result.

3 Spoon the mixture into the paper liners and bake in a—preheated oven, 400°F, for 15–20 minutes. Let cool a little and serve.

Eating an **apple** with your lunch, or as an afternoon snack, can help stop sugar cravings. Research has also found that the fruit contains **anticarcinogenic properties**, so all the more reason for you to enjoy an apple a day.

nutritional values per serving | Cals **143 (603 kj)** | Protein **4 g** | Carb **24 g** | Fat **4 g**

banana bread

preparation: 15 minutes | **cooking:** 1–1¼ hours | **serves:** 12

scant ⅓ cup polyunsaturated margarine, plus extra for greasing

½ cup brown sugar

2 large eggs, beaten

3 large bananas, coarsely mashed

scant ½ cup dates, coarsely chopped

½ cup walnuts, chopped

generous ¾ cup buttermilk

1½ cups all-purpose whole wheat flour

1 teaspoon baking soda

1 Lightly grease and line a 1¾-lb loaf pan. In a large bowl, beat the margarine and sugar together until light and fluffy. Beat in the eggs, a little at a time, then stir in the bananas, dates, walnuts, and buttermilk. Gently fold in the flour and baking soda.

2 Spoon into the prepared pan, then bake in a preheated oven, 350°F, for about 1–1¼ hours until a skewer comes out clean when inserted. Let cool, then serve.

nutritional values per serving | Cals **238 (1000 kj)** | Protein **6 g** | Carb **34 g** | Fat **10 g**

coconut cookies

preparation: 15 minutes, plus chilling | **cooking:** 7–8 minutes | **makes:** 18

½ cup cornmeal

¼ cup all-purpose whole wheat flour

½ teaspoon baking powder

scant ⅔ cup confectioners' sugar

¼ cup butter, cubed and chilled

scant ½ cup dry unsweetened coconut

few drops of vanilla extract

2 egg yolks

2 oz semisweet chocolate

1 Line 2 cookie sheets with parchment paper. In a bowl, stir the cornmeal, flour, baking powder, and sugar together, then cut in the butter using your fingertips until the mixture resembles fine breadcrumbs. Stir through the coconut, then the vanilla extract and egg yolks to combine. Form into a firm dough, then roll into a sausage 2 inches in diameter. Wrap in foil and chill in the refrigerator for 30 minutes.

2 Cut the dough "sausage" into 18 slices and place well apart on the prepared cookie sheets. Bake in a preheated oven, 350°F, for 7–8 minutes until golden. Let cool on the cookie sheets.

3 Break the chocolate into pieces and put them in a heatproof bowl over a pan of lightly simmering water until the chocolate has melted. Drizzle over the cookies using the back of a spoon.

nutritional values per serving | Cals **97 (407 kj)** | Protein **1 g** | Carb **11 g** | Fat **6 g**

fruit and nut bars

preparation: 10 minutes | **cooking:** 15 minutes | **makes:** 8

scant ½ cup butter or polyunsaturated margarine, plus extra for greasing

4 tablespoons maple syrup

2 tablespoons light brown sugar

2 cups jumbo oats

generous ½ cup oatmeal

⅓ cup chopped mixed nuts

generous ¾ cup mixed dried fruit (such as figs, dates, no-soak apricots, and cranberries), chopped

2 tablespoons sunflower seeds

1 Lightly grease and base-line an 8-inch square, nonstick baking pan. In a pan, melt the butter or margarine, syrup, and sugar together. Stir in all the remaining ingredients, except the sunflower seeds, then press the mixture into the prepared pan.

2 Sprinkle over the sunflower seeds, then bake in a preheated oven, 400°F, for 15 minutes until golden. Mark into 8 bars. Let cool, then serve.

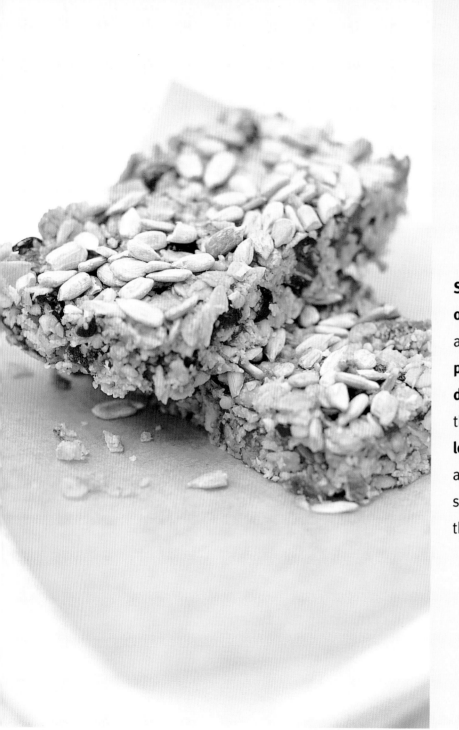

Sunflower seeds are **rich in omega-3 and omega-6** fatty acids, which can help **protect against heart disease**. They also contain the unsaturated fats that **lower blood cholesterol**, so all in all, they're a bit of a super seed! Try sprinkling them over salads or cereal.

nutritional values per serving | Cals **368 (1542 kj)** | Protein **6 g** | Carb **46 g** | Fat **19 g**

mixed seed rolls

preparation: 20 minutes, plus proving | **cooking:** 20 minutes | **makes:** 8

2⅔ cups whole wheat flour, plus extra for dusting

pinch of salt

1 tablespoon active dry yeast

3½ oz mixed seeds (such as sesame, sunflower, and pumpkin)

2 tablespoons clear honey

1 cup hand-hot water

oil, for oiling

1 In a large bowl, mix the flour, salt, yeast, and the mixed seeds (reserve 1 tablespoon) together. Stir half the honey into the water, then pour into the flour and form into a soft dough.

2 Tip out on to a lightly floured counter and knead for about 5 minutes. Place in a lightly oiled bowl, cover with a damp cloth, and let prove in a warm place until doubled in size.

3 Reknead the dough for 5 minutes, then divide into 8 pieces. Knead to form rolls, then place on a cookie sheet, cover, and let prove again until doubled in size.

4 Brush over the remaining honey and sprinkle over the reserved seeds. Bake in a preheated oven, 400°F, for 20 minutes until the rolls are golden and sound hollow when tapped.

nutritional values per serving | Cals **270 (1140 kJ)** | Protein **10 g** | Carb **44 g** | Fat **7 g**

rye bread

preparation: 20 minutes, plus proving | **cooking:** 30–35 minutes | **makes:** 2 x 1 lb (500 g) loaves

3 cups white bread flour, plus extra for dusting

3 cups rye flour

2 tablespoons active dry yeast

2 teaspoons caraway seeds

1 teaspoon salt

4 tablespoons oil, plus extra for oiling

1 tablespoon clear honey

4 tablespoons lowfat plain yogurt

2¼ cups tepid water

1 In a large bowl, mix the flours, yeast, caraway seeds, and salt together. Stir the remaining ingredients into the water, then gradually stir into the flour mixture to form a soft dough.

2 Tip out on to a lightly floured counter and knead for 5 minutes until smooth. Place in a lightly oiled bowl, cover with a damp cloth, and let prove in a warm place for 1 hour until doubled in size.

3 Reknead the dough, divide into 2 pieces, and shape each into an oval loaf. Place the loaves on lightly floured cookie sheets, cover with a damp cloth, and let prove again until doubled in size.

4 Slash the tops of the loaves a few times with a sharp knife, then bake in a preheated oven, 400°F, for 30–35 minutes until golden and sounding hollow when tapped. Let cool on a cooling rack, then serve.

nutritional values per serving | Cals **152 (646 kj)** | Protein **4 g** | Carb **30 g** | Fat **3 g**

rustic nutty seed loaf

preparation: 15 minutes, plus proving | **cooking:** 30–35 minutes | **makes:** 1 large loaf

2¾ cups whole wheat flour, plus extra for dusting

1 teaspoon salt

3½ oz mixed seeds (such as pumpkin, sunflower, and poppy)

2 tablespoons bulgur wheat

1½ tablespoons active dry yeast

⅓ cup mixed nuts (such as hazelnuts and walnuts), chopped

6 scallions, sliced

½ cup Parmesan cheese, freshly grated

1 tablespoon clear honey

1¼ cups warm water

oil, for oiling

1 In a large bowl, mix all the ingredients, except the honey and water, together. Blend the honey with the water, then stir into the flour mix and form into a dough.

2 Tip out on to a lightly floured counter and knead for 5 minutes until smooth. Place in a lightly oiled bowl, cover with a damp cloth, and let prove in a warm place for 2 hours until doubled in size.

3 Reknead the dough, shape into a circle, and place on a cookie sheet. Cover with a damp cloth and let prove again for 1 hour. Bake in a preheated oven, 425°F, for 30–35 minutes until it sounds hollow when tapped.

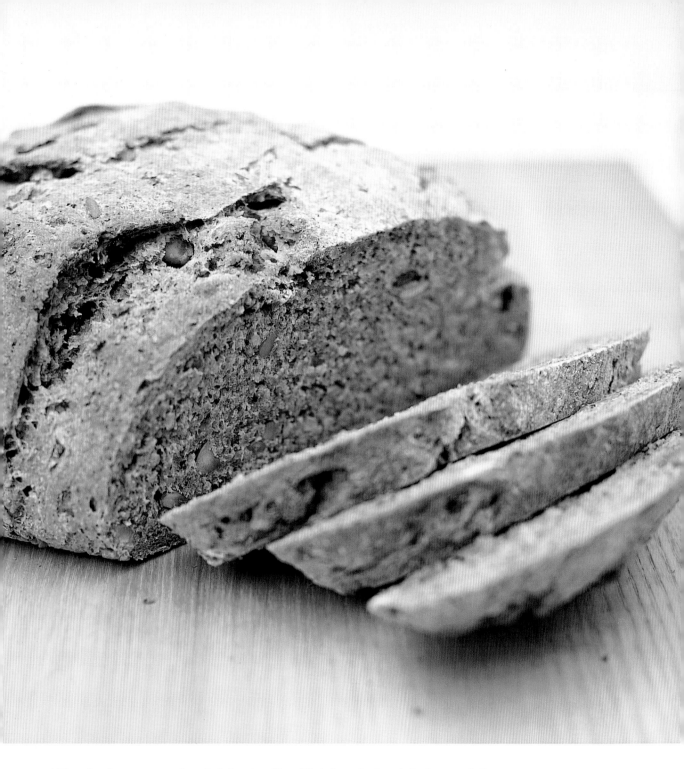

nutritional values per serving | Cals **165** **(697 kJ)** | Protein **8 g** | Carb **23 g** | Fat **7 g**

orange and golden raisin biscuits

preparation: 20 minutes | **cooking:** about 10 minutes | **makes:** 12

generous ¾ cup self-rising flour, plus extra for dusting

scant ⅔ cup whole wheat self-rising flour

2 teaspoons baking powder

¼ cup butter, cubed and chilled

generous ¼ cup golden raisins

1 tablespoon superfine sugar

grated rind of 1 orange

1 egg

about ½ cup milk

to serve

cream cheese

fresh strawberries (optional)

1 Sift the flours and baking powder into a large bowl, tipping any bran in the strainer back into the bowl. Cut in the butter using your fingers until the mix resembles fine breadcrumbs, then stir in the golden raisins, sugar, and orange rind.

2 Break the egg into a measuring cup and beat with a fork. Make up to ⅔ cup with milk, then pour into the flour mixture and bring together to form a soft dough, adding a little extra milk if the dough is too dry.

3 Press gently into a ½-inch thick circle. Stamp out about 12 biscuits, place on lightly floured cookie sheets, and brush with a little milk. Bake in a preheated oven, 425°F, for about 10 minutes, until risen and golden.

4 Let the biscuits cool on a cooling rack, then serve that day to enjoy them at their best. Serve with a little cream cheese and fresh strawberries, if liked, to bring the overall GI down.

nutritional values per serving | Cals **120 (505 kJ)** | Protein **3 g** | Carb **18 g** | Fat **4 g**

sesame seed oatcakes

preparation: 10 minutes | **cooking:** about 10 minutes | **makes:** about 12

generous 1 cup oatmeal

1 tablespoon sesame seeds

pinch of salt

pinch of baking soda

1 tablespoon olive oil

2–3 tablespoons hot water

flour, for dusting

1 In a bowl, mix all the ingredients together to form a firm dough, adding a little extra water if necessary. The mixture will be very crumbly, so just keep pressing it back together.

2 Roll the mixture out on a lightly floured counter as thinly as you can. Cut out triangles or 3-inch circles and place on cookie sheets. Bake in a preheated oven, 350°F, for about 10 minutes until golden and firm. Let cool on a cooling rack.

nutritional values per serving | Cals **79 (330 kj)** | Protein **2 g** | Carb **11 g** | Fat **3 g**

pesto and sesame seed pastry twists

preparation: 10 minutes | **cooking:** 8–10 minutes | **makes:** 15

8 oz Short-Crust Pastry (see page 94)

flour, for dusting

2 tablespoons pesto

2 tablespoons milk or a little beaten egg

2 tablespoons sesame seeds

1 Roll the pie dough out on a lightly floured counter to a 10-inch square. Spoon over the pesto and smooth out, then cut the pie dough into 15 strips.

2 Twist the strips and place on a cookie sheet. Brush with a little milk or egg and sprinkle over the sesame seeds. Bake in a preheated oven, 400°F, for 8–10 minutes until golden.

nutritional values per serving | Cals **94 (390 kj)** | Protein **2 g** | Carb **8 g** | Fat **6 g**

Parmesan and Caerphilly crackers

preparation: 10 minutes, plus chilling | **cooking:** 10–12 minutes | **makes:** 20

¾ cup all-purpose whole wheat flour

scant ⅓ cup butter, cubed and chilled, or polyunsaturated margarine, cut into pieces

2 tablespoons polenta

3½ oz Caerphilly cheese, or other crumbly cheese, crumbled

½ cup Parmesan cheese, freshly grated

generous ¼ cup no-soak dried apricots

1 egg yolk

cheese or fresh fruit (such as apples or pears), to serve

1 Sift the flour into a bowl and cut in the butter or margarine with your fingertips until the mixture resembles fine breadcrumbs. Stir in the polenta, cheeses, and apricots, then add the egg yolk and bring the mixture together to form a ball. It will be very crumbly, so just keep pressing it back together.

2 Roll the ball into a sausage about 2 inches in diameter, wrap in foil, then chill in the refrigerator for 30 minutes. Cut the dough "sausage" into 20 slices, place on cookie sheets, and bake in a preheated oven, 400°F, for 10–12 minutes until golden. Let cool, then serve with cheese or fresh fruit to keep the GI down.

nutritional values per serving | Cals **90 (373 kj)** | Protein **3 g** | Carb **6 g** | Fat **6 g**

index

acknowledgments

Executive Editor Nicola Hill
Editor Charlotte Wilson
Executive Art Editor Joanna MacGregor
Designer Ginny Zeal
Senior Production Controller Martin Croshaw
Picture Researcher Jennifer Veall

Food Stylist Joss Herd
Photographer Gareth Sambidge